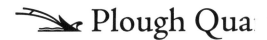 **Plough Qua**

BREAKING GROUND FOR A RENEWED WORLD

Winter 2018, Number 15

Feature: The Tech Issue

Views and Reviews

Artists: Pieter Bruegel the Elder, Jack Baumgartner, Nicholas Roerich, Rachel Newling, Kay Polk, Suellen McCrary, Stephen Scott Young, Jie Wei Zhou, Kiéra Malone, Torkel Pettersson, Mari Rast, Albrecht Dürer, René Magritte
Cover: Kyle T. Webster

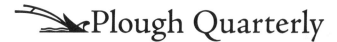

Plough Quarterly

WWW.PLOUGH.COM

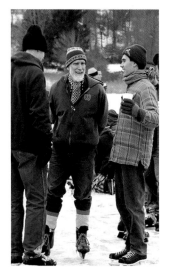

Meet the community behind *Plough*.

Plough Quarterly is published by the Bruderhof, an international community of families and singles seeking to follow Jesus together. Members of the Bruderhof are committed to a way of radical discipleship in the spirit of the Sermon on the Mount. Inspired by the first church in Jerusalem (Acts 2 and 4), they renounce private property and share everything in common in a life of nonviolence, justice, and service to neighbors near and far. The community includes people from a wide range of backgrounds. There are twenty-three Bruderhof settlements in both rural and urban locations in the United States, England, Germany, Australia, and Paraguay, with around 2,900 people in all.

To learn more or arrange a visit, see the community's website at *bruderhof.com.*

Plough Quarterly features original stories, ideas, and culture to inspire everyday faith and action. Starting from the conviction that the teachings and example of Jesus can transform and renew our world, we aim to apply them to all aspects of life, seeking common ground with all people of goodwill regardless of creed. The goal of *Plough Quarterly* is to build a living network of readers, contributors, and practitioners so that, in the words of Hebrews, we may "spur one another on toward love and good deeds."

Plough Quarterly includes contributions that we believe are worthy of our readers' consideration, whether or not we fully agree with them. Views expressed by contributors are their own and do not necessarily reflect the editorial position of *Plough* or of the Bruderhof communities.

Editors: Peter Mommsen, Veery Huleatt, Sam Hine. Art director: Emily Alexander. Managing editor: Shana Burleson.
Contributing editors: Maureen Swinger, Susannah Black, Bernard Hibbs, Chungyon Won, Charles Moore.
Founding Editor: Eberhard Arnold (1883–1935).
Plough Quarterly No. 15: Technology
Published by Plough Publishing House, ISBN 978-0-87486-040-5
Copyright © 2018 by Plough Publishing House. All rights reserved.

Editorial Office
PO Box 398
Walden, NY 12586
T: 845.572.3455
info@plough.com

Subscriber Services
PO Box 345
Congers, NY 10920-0345
T: 800.521.8011
subscriptions@plough.com

United Kingdom
Brightling Road
Robertsbridge
TN32 5DR
T: +44(0)1580.883.344

Australia
4188 Gwydir Highway
Elsmore, NSW
2360 Australia
T: +61(0)2.6723.2213

Plough Quarterly (ISSN 2372-2584) is published quarterly by Plough Publishing House, PO Box 398, Walden, NY 12586.
Individual subscription $32 per year in the United States; Canada add $8, other countries add $16.
Periodicals postage paid at Walden, NY 12586 and at additional mailing offices.
POSTMASTER: Send address changes to *Plough Quarterly*, PO Box 345, Congers, NY 10920-0345.

STATEMENT OF OWNERSHIP, MANAGEMENT, AND CIRCULATION (Required by 39 U.S.C. 3685) 1. Title of publication: Plough Quarterly. 2. Publication No: 0001-6584. 3. Date of filing: October 1, 2017. 4. Frequency of issue: Quarterly. 5. Number of issues published annually: 4. 6. Annual subscription price: $32.00. 7. Complete mailing address of known office of publication: Plough Quarterly, P.O. Box 398, Walden, NY 12586. 8. Same. 9. Publisher: Plough Publishing House, same address. Editor: Peter Mommsen, same address. Managing Editor: Sam Hine, same address. 10. Owner: Church Communities Foundation, 2032 Rte 213, Rifton, NY 12471. 11. Known bondholders, mortgages, and other securities: None. 12. The purpose, function, and nonprofit status of this organization and the exempt status for federal income tax purposes have not changed during preceding 12 months. 13. Publication Title: Plough Quarterly. 14. Issue date for circulation data below: Fall 2016–Summer 2017. 15. Extent and nature of circulation: Average No. copies of each issue during preceding 12 months: A. Total number of copies (net press run)—12,535. B.1. Mailed outside-county paid subscriptions: 7,108. B.2. Mailed in-county paid subscriptions: 0. B.3. Paid distribution outside the mails including sales through dealers and carriers, street vendors, counter sales, and other non-USPS paid distribution: 217. B.4. Other classes mailed through the USPS: 0. C. Total paid distribution: 7,325. D.1. Free distribution by mail: Outside-county—799. D.2. In-county—0. D.3. Other classes mailed through the USPS—0. Free distribution outside the mail—3,335. E. Total free distribution: 4,134. F. Total Distribution: 11,458. G. Copies not distributed: 1,077. H. Total: 12,535. I. Percent paid—63.92%. Actual No. copies of single issue published nearest to filing date: A. 14,000. B.1. 8,155. B.2. 0. B.3. 239. B.4. 0. C. 8,394. D.1. 892. D.2. 0. D.3. 0. D.4. 3,335. E. 4,227. F. 12,621. G. 1,379. H. 14,000. I. 66.51%. Electronic copy circulation: Average No. copies of each issue during preceding 12 months: A. Total No. Electronic Copies: 270. B. Total paid print copies plus paid electronic copies: 7,595. C. Total print distribution plus paid electronic copies: 11,728. D. Percent paid: 64.76%. Actual No. copies of single issue published nearest to filing date: A. 315. B. 8,709. C. 12,936. D. 67.32%. 17. Publication of Statement of Ownership: Winter 2018. 18. I certify that the statements made by me above are correct and complete. Sam Hine, Editor, October 1, 2017.

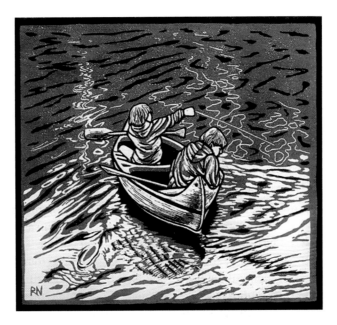

The Joys of Tech Asceticism
On Staying Human

PETER MOMMSEN

Dear Reader,

Elon Musk, the man who started four billion-dollar tech companies, is worried that computers are on course to kill us. As he told an audience at MIT in 2014, "With artificial intelligence, we are summoning the demon." In his nightmare, a future superintelligent machine will outwit and then eliminate humankind. Accordingly, Musk is working on plans to colonize other planets in case we, or the artificial minds we create, make human survival on Earth impossible.

Is Musk paranoid? Inconveniently for his detractors, he's no agrarian crank, and his concern about artificial intelligence (AI) is shared by people as diverse as Henry Kissinger, Stephen Hawking, and Bill Gates. According to their line of thinking, AI may soon rank among the threats to humanity's survival alongside nuclear war and biological terrorism.

These anxieties exemplify a wider shift. For a generation, a utopian glow has hung around Silicon Valley and all its works. Now that glow is fading fast. Critics on both the political left and right assail the monopolistic power wielded by Google, Apple, Facebook, and Amazon. From Washington to Brussels, Big Tech's gospel of libertarian capitalism twinned with libertarian morality has worn out its welcome. Once upon a time, Mark Zuckerberg's motto of "move fast and break things" sounded innocently boyish; now it seems to sum up all too well the menace of machines to humans. Already, robots are replacing workers at an alarming rate.

Stung by the backlash, technophiles point to technology's achievements: What about

Rachel Newling, *Waiting for Fish*, linocut

the myriad ways it has reduced misery and enhanced the quality of human life? What about the printing press and electric lights and antibiotics and instant global communication and cancer drugs?

It's a valid point. No one, from Apple engineers to Amish farmers, wants to return to a tech-free world of fifty-percent child mortality and surgery without anesthetics. The urge to invent and use tools, to pioneer new frontiers of ingenuity, is part and parcel of being human and has brought astounding benefits. To Christian eyes, this inborn inventiveness reflects the Creator himself and corresponds to the task that he gave to humankind in the Book of Genesis: to be master and steward of creation on his behalf.

> **Nobody wants to return to a tech-free world of surgery without anesthetics.**

Still, this doesn't provide much reassurance when new technologies are rewiring the brains of today's children and will likely soon be used to edit the genomes of those to be born. We're living in a radically new situation. How do we stay human?

We can start by taking Elon Musk literally: "With artificial intelligence, we are summoning the demon." Whatever Musk meant by these words, they fit with strange precision into the New Testament's view of reality. As the biblical writers saw it, the major social systems that shape human communities are not merely impersonal. Rather, such systems – which include the state, religious institutions, and today surely also the technological structures that govern modern life – operate under the influence of distinct spiritual forces. The New Testament uses a range of names for these spiritual powers, among them *daimonia:* "demons." It's an awkward word. Yet in view of Silicon Valley's fascination with transhumanism and rationalist ideology (pages 20 and 26), to speak here of demons may be all too apt.

Recognizing that uncanny forces lurk within technological structures doesn't require us to flee the Information Age. But it does mean Christians must stop pretending that technological products are just neutral tools (page 49).

The example of social media proves the point. Sean Parker, a founding president of Facebook, recently admitted in an interview that Facebook was designed to be addictive, adding, "God only knows what it's doing to our children's brains." Actually, even without special revelation, we already know: studies of teenagers show a strong correlation between heavy social media use and anxiety, depression, and suicide, as documented by Jean Twenge in the *Atlantic*. This is not what human flourishing looks like.

For Christians, mental health risks are not the only concern. In Christ's service we are pledged to spend all our energies doing good to our flesh-and-blood neighbors, building up a living symbol of his coming kingdom here on earth in community with others (page 44). This calling is incompatible with spending hours in thrall to a screen, not-quite-voluntarily chasing the next dopamine hit.

More often than not, then, the best social media policy is also the simplest: abstinence. Even those with strong reasons to post and tweet – keep up the good work, *Plough* social media editors! – need to set themselves firm guidelines. *Plough*'s house rule, for example, is to avoid social media outside of work hours, especially since many of us have young children at home. (The bonus family time can be spent in the great outdoors, reading or singing together – or building harps, as Maureen Swinger describes on page 18.)

When it comes to children, tech abstinence is hardly a fringe idea. Steve Jobs famously refused to give his kids tablets or smartphones; as Johann Christoph Arnold writes, the abundant benefits of a screen-free childhood are widely acknowledged (page 34). More ominously, evidence is mounting of the long-term damage caused by internet pornography. In the face of this insidious horror, deciding to keep one's children offline is not a tough call. Yes, it's easier said than done, and may require changes to lifestyle and spending patterns, switching schools, or even moving. But to a Christian parent, does any other value out-weigh the soul of a child? And life offline can be fun (pages 55 and 58).

The joys of abstinence need not be restricted to new technologies, either. Forty years have passed since the advertising executive Jerry Mander provoked a national debate with his book *Four Arguments for the Elimination of Television,* and all of his arguments remain as compelling as ever. Here's to the day when having a TV in the family living room will be as disreputable as having a cigarette-butt-strewn ashtray is now.

Voice such ideas, and sooner or later you'll be called a Luddite. Rather than reject the label, then, perhaps we should rehabilitate it. The original Luddites of nineteenth-century England didn't risk the gallows out of senti-mental technophobia. They were working-class weavers who rose in protest when a new invention, the frame loom, threatened their livelihoods and communities. While it's true they smashed machinery, their real opponent was the greed of textile barons who stood to make a fortune by putting them out of work. In a society warped by technological consum-erism, a bracing dose of nonviolent Luddite rebellion might be just what we need.

The Luddites' message was straightforward:

people come before machines and profits. Surely that's a slogan that both social-justice progressives and traditional conservatives can make their own. This is the truth at the centerpiece of Pope Francis's encyclical *Laudato si'*. Economists may mutter about what they call the Luddite fallacy, but the "people first" principle stands.

Jesus, too, taught that the welfare of human beings is paramount, trumping both economic efficiency and religious precepts. We can't mine his words in the Gospels for proof texts on the newest technologies. But we can take seriously his teaching on an old technology: money. The technology of money was as essential to the functioning of society in the first century as it is in the twenty-first. Jesus never prohibited his followers from using it. But he came uncomfortably close, describing money not as a mere tool but as a personified false god boasting its own Aramaic name: "No one can serve two masters. . . . You cannot serve God and Mammon" (Luke 16:13).

The Luddites' message was straightforward: people come before machines and profits.

The same either-or clarity will be necessary as we hurtle toward an increasingly techno-logical future. Technological asceticism on its own won't solve society-wide dilemmas, much less save our species from extinction. Its function is more basic: to help us maintain the spiritual independence needed to tackle these challenges. Like any other kind of asceticism, it requires regular practice. But the reward is worth having: the prize of staying human.

Warm greetings,

Peter

Peter Mommsen
Editor

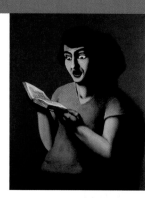

René Magritte, *The Submissive Reader*

Winners or Losers?

On Peter Mommsen's "The Church We Need Now," Autumn 2017: Peter Mommsen claims that the Anabaptist Reformation not only "matters," but "won," and tells why. He knows that it is very unbaptistic to make extravagant claims that "we're number one." But he does point to three reforms, neglected or disdained when Anabaptist movements were formed in the sixteenth century, whose teachings and practices made them look like "losers," or made them to be losers when the hangmen from the other four versions [of the Reformation: Lutheran, Calvinist, Anglican, and Catholic] defeated or even killed them. . . .

Is this boasting? At the end, Mommsen acknowledges some specialty weaknesses that do not deserve to be praised or copied. This cluster of Protestants did not "win," as Mommsen's article claims. But its witness is heard and its effects are still seen where religious freedom, nonviolence, and community are present in fresh ways.

Martin E. Marty, Chicago, IL
From the blog Sightings: Religion and Public Life, *November 27, 2017*

Thirty years ago I wrote a book (*Theology in Postliberal Perspective*) suggesting that these three concepts – freedom of belief, pacifist nonviolence, and a communal ethos of mutual aid and support – were the central features of Anabaptist spirituality and practice, on which a church of the future could thrive. That book found much better reception outside of the Anabaptist churches than within, so I am quite heartened to read this essay by Peter Mommsen today!

Daniel Liechty, Normal, IL

The Church's Politics

On George Weigel's "Re-Forming the Church," Autumn 2017: I am in agreement with George Weigel's understanding of what makes authentic reform in the Church. I disagree, however, with his understanding of the example that he gives: the Catholic Church's affirmation of religious freedom at Vatican II. According to Weigel, Vatican II's declaration on religious liberty, *Dignitatis humanae,* represented a rejection of the "thesis" that the best arrangement of church–state relations would be an "establishment" of the Church, in which temporal power recognized the authority of spiritual power and the truth of the Faith. His has been the conventional reading of *Dignitatis humanae.* But the document itself explicitly excludes such a reading, stating that it "leaves untouched traditional Catholic doctrine on the moral duty of men and societies toward the true religion and toward the one Church of Christ." As recent interpreters such as Thomas Pink have demonstrated, Vatican II's affirmation of religious freedom is fully consistent with the soul–body model of Church–state relations taught by popes such as Leo XIII.

Yes, what the Church needs most are witnesses on fire with the love of Christ. But such persons should be the first to recognize that loving Christ means ordering all things to him, including political societies. All political action is concerned with realizing the good, and things can only be adequately judged good with respect to the highest good and last end. It is therefore impossible for political action to be "neutral" with respect to the last end: either it will order itself to the true good in God, or to a false idol.

Weigel claims that establishment leads to secularization, whereas disestablishment leads to the Church prospering and growing. But it is hard to see how this claim holds up with a view to current trends. Secularization has only accelerated more and more since European nations gave up establishment. And even the United States, which once seemed exceptional in that regard, now seems to be catching up with Europe.

Pater Edmund Waldstein, O.Cist., Austria

George Weigel responds: Thesis–hypothesis was, as I understand it, not a matter of doctrine but of theological opinion, so my claims about *Dignitatis humanae* are not affected by the citation from the document quoted by Father Waldstein.

As for establishment contributing to the decline of Christianity under conditions of modernity, I offer Father Waldstein the examples of Spain, Portugal, Ireland, and Quebec, where the Church leaned heavily on state support in one form or another – and the faith collapsed within two generations when the tidal wave of cultural sludge let loose in the Sixties overwhelmed those societies. Poland, where the bishops are too publicly identified today with one political party, might ponder this experience.

I would be interested to know if Father Waldstein believes (along with Father John Courtney Murray, SJ, one of the intellectual architects of *Dignitatis humanae*) that the natural law can provide a public moral grammar for the ordering of societies, one that can function amidst confessional differences. That would seem at least one possible alternative to either states becoming theological actors again, or the impending dictatorship of relativism of which Pope Benedict XVI warned.

As Father Waldstein may know, I am fully committed to the New Evangelization, a position I laid out in *Evangelical Catholicism: Deep Reform in the 21st-Century Church*. But having President Donald Trump publicly recognize Jesus Christ as King of the United States of America hardly strikes me as something that would advance the cause of the gospel.

Last Christians in Iraq?

On Andreas Knapp's "The Last of the First Christians," Autumn 2017: After working in Iraq over the past fifteen years with Christian Peacemaker Teams, I am always glad when people voice their concern about the people of Iraq. I was touched by the love Andreas Knapp showed in dropping his work to accompany his new refugee friend, Yousif, back to northern Iraq.

I have difficulty, though, with some of Knapp's statements. Yes, large numbers of jihadists from all over the Muslim world came to Iraq in response to the 2003 US invasion, and threatened some Christians because they aligned them with the "Christian" United States, but Iraqi Christians were not their main target. They bombed mosques, especially Shia mosques, as well as churches. Other targets included sites connected with US forces and the Iraqi police forces as well as general public sites. The goal was to destabilize society and get rid of US occupation. In some places Muslims did take advantage of the chaos to drive out or even kill their Christian neighbors. But there was never a large-scale jihad or genocide against Christians.

What Knapp writes about protection money happened in some places, particularly in Mosul, but was not widespread elsewhere. I related to many Christians and church groups in southern and central Iraq, but had never heard of a Christian tax until ISIS took over Mosul and enacted it more widely there. ISIS gave most Christians in Mosul the choice of leaving the city or paying the tax.

Since the US invasion, criminal gangs in Iraq have kidnapped and sometimes killed many Christians for the purpose of extracting money, but not proportionally more than Muslims.

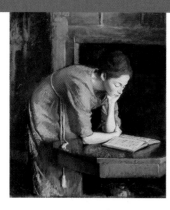

Image from readingandart.blogspot.com

Aaron Shikler, *Woman Reading (The Artist's Wife)*

When ISIS occupied parts of Iraq in 2014, it destroyed or took over a number of Christian churches. Violence against Christians increased. There were some Christians killed by ISIS, but in general Shia Muslims and Yezidi people fared worse. The Yezidis were the most systematically targeted, to the degree that this could be labeled "genocide." That doesn't make the times Christians were killed, threatened, or forced from their homes any less horrible, or lessen the witness of those Christians who were killed for refusing to deny their faith. But there hasn't been, and isn't currently, a widespread genocide against Christians or an attempt to stamp out Christianity in Iraq.

In spite of my concerns with this article, my hope for readers of Knapp's book is that they will come away with more compassion for displaced Christians, Muslims, and Yezidis from Iraq (and for displaced Christians from Palestine, and the Muslim Rohingya people currently being killed, abused, and displaced), and become more committed to witness against such wars of aggression that led to the suffering Knapp describes. *Peggy Gish, Athens, OH*

Doing the Little Things Better

On Claudio Oliver's "The Unplanned Church," Autumn 2017: Claudio, your life and community continue to shape our own here in Kentucky as we, too, seek to be more faithful to our human vocation. I write this looking out over beds of winter greens, watching the chickens dig out the flesh from pumpkins, as songbirds flit from tree to tree, easily visible in the bare branches. We are surrounded by beauty and goodness – gifts of a generous and loving Creator. And they continually ask me: "Are my neighbors sharing in this goodness?" "What more can we do to share in this goodness together?" *Sean Gladding, Lexington, KY*

I love thinking of a sense of reduction as God's call – as a church, when do we do too much? How can we simplify and do the little things better – welcoming neighbors, responding to needs, listening, and loving?
Nathan Hill, New Carrolton, MD

Both Old and Young

On Jin Kim's "Time for a New Reformation," Autumn 2017: I am thankful for the witness of the Church of All Nations, and the discernment that Pastor Kim has been given regarding the spirit of the times. Indeed, the church in America is suffering from an identity crisis. Have we grown tired and weary of trying to characterize and measure ourselves by a standard apart from Christ, and him crucified? No wonder so many leave the church: we are shaped by a culture that demands our own comforts and rights, and then we build churches that attempt to cater to these egoisms.

I'm grateful to be experiencing the kind of transformation Pastor Jin describes here in Chattanooga, as part of the New City East Lake community. We are seeking to be the body of Christ in an urban neighborhood that has historically been torn apart by the racial tensions and divisions typical of the American South. In addition, recent decades have brought a large contingency of Latino neighbors as well, adding another layer of cultural complexity. Our call is to witness to God's promised kingdom as a worshiping community reconciled across these cultural lines by living and working together in East Lake.

It is not without much struggle, pain, and brokenness, but we are also seeking to be rooted in Jesus and the tradition of "radical faithfulness to the God of Israel." I thank God for communities like CAN and the Bruderhof for keeping the fire burning.

Joshua Livingston, Chattanooga, TN

I wholeheartedly agree with your assertion that young people are searching for vocation, healthy relationships, community, concreteness in a virtual world, and authentic faith. But it's not just young people – don't count us gray heads out! In addition to being multiethnic, a vibrant Christian community must be multigenerational. Having said that, I admire what you are doing, especially that you are doing it within the framework of a mainline denomination! You have inspired me. But if I don't find a framework, I might have to start something.

Al Owski, Commerce Township, MI

Jin Kim responds: I believe that a vibrant congregation will reflect the diversity of the surrounding context, including generational diversity. At Church of All Nations we are truly blessed to have every generation represented in our congregational life. The younger generation shows honor and affection to the older, the older generation passes on hard-earned wisdom to the younger, and those in the middle serve as pillars of support to the very young and old.

Where Is Your Hope?

On Rowan Williams's "The Two Ways," Autumn 2017: There is a close relationship between loyalty and hope. Dr. Williams has helpfully depicted the remarkable shift in allegiance that marked out the early Christian church. Jews and Greeks, Romans and Syrians, and many more surrendered their tribal and national and familial and religious allegiances and embraced, through baptism, a new loyalty to Christ. It may be better to say that through faith and baptism they *were embraced* into a new loyalty. In any

event, it was indeed a new and, as Dr. Williams reminds us, an unprecedented challenge to the loyalty systems of the time.

This new loyalty to Christ as Lord carried with it a new hope. What else but hope could embolden a young Roman woman to seek out the Lord's Supper at risk of life itself? What else but hope could take "death-cell philosophy" and fill it with gospel joy? If by faith and baptism God embraced these Romans into Christ, adopting them as children, and granting them citizenship in heaven, then theirs was the happy hope of "an inheritance that is imperishable, undefiled, and unfading, kept in heaven . . . ," for they were guarded by God's power (1 Pet. 1:4–5). Loyalty to Christ and hopefulness in Christ cannot be separated.

But that carries a troubling implication: If loyalty to Christ and hopefulness go together, then what does it mean when hope deteriorates? Imagine a Christian community that is captivated by (for instance) the state: sometimes distrustful and hostile toward it, other times fiercely defensive of it, but always fascinated by it. Imagine further that over time the Christian community's frustration and contentment rises and falls on the political cycle. Might this imply that the Christian community had atrophied in its hope? Could it be that such patterns implied that the state had become the object of hope rather than the Lord who embraced the church? And if this be granted, might it be that an atrophied hope implies a deteriorated loyalty to Christ?

I imagine a young Roman slave girl, walking early in the morning through the streets of Ephesus, eager to join her true family in the celebration of her Lord's Supper. She is defying her state, but she does not hate Caesar. She loves Christ. And it is her love for Christ – her loyalty to the Lord who gave her true citizenship at

(Continued on page 12)

Return to Sender in Wittenberg

The peace pilgrims by the statue of Philipp Melanchthon in the main square of Wittenberg

After a ten-day bicycle pilgrimage from Augsburg to Wittenberg, Article XVI of the Augsburg Confession is finally back on its author's desk.

Twenty cyclists recently traveled through wind and weather, covering the three hundred and seventy miles between Augsburg and Wittenburg. They arrived in Wittenburg on September 10, just in time for the concluding worship service of the Reformation World Fair. Their mission? To return the Augsburg Confession's Article XVI to its place of origin. "We're returning something that should never have left the gates of Wittenberg," said Thomas Nauerth, the campaign's initiator, organizer, and navigator.

The Augsburg Confession, a central Reformation confession of faith, was authored by Philipp Melanchthon in 1530. The document still belongs to the official confessions of a range of Protestant churches and, because of this official status, many pastors and church deacons are duty-bound to uphold it. Article XVI states ". . . that lawful civil ordinances

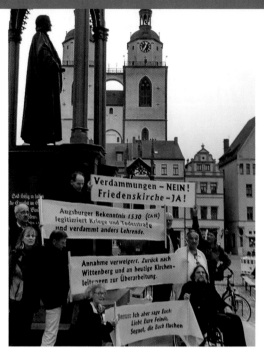

Image from Vorarlberger KirchenBlatt 21. September 2017

are good works of God, and that *it is right for Christians* to bear civil office, to sit as judges, to judge matters by the Imperial and other existing laws, to *award just punishments, to engage in just wars, to serve as soldiers,* to make legal contracts, to hold property, to make oath when required. . . . They *condemn the*

The Forgotten Martyrs of World War I

In a historic week for war dissenters of all stripes, the pacifists of World War I were recognized at the Remembering Muted Voices Symposium, which took place in October at the National World War I Museum in Kansas City. Andrew Bolton, the conference organizer, was inspired by the story of Hutterite conscientious objectors Joseph and Michael Hofer, who died as a result of mistreatment in Alcatraz Federal Penitentiary and Fort Leavenworth Disciplinary Barracks, where

they were imprisoned for their pacifist convictions. (See Duane Stoltzfus's "The Martyrs of Alcatraz," *Plough* no. 1.)

The event sponsors were diverse, including the American Friends Service Committee, the War Resisters League, the American Civil Liberties Union, and the Mennonite Central Committee. At the conference's conclusion, a stone in remembrance of Joseph and Michael Hofer was unveiled. It will be placed in the Walk of Honor at the foot of the Liberty

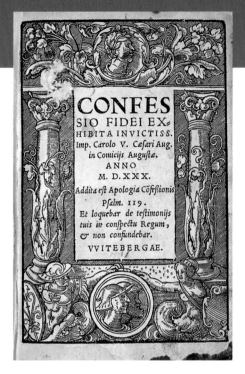

The title page of the Augsburg Confession presented on June 25, 1530 to Emperor Charles V

Anabaptists who forbid these civil offices to Christians" (author's emphasis).

The cyclists' proposal? It's time for Article XVI to go. The International Fellowship of Reconciliation (IFOR), of which Nauerth is a member, has campaigned against injustice and war since 1914. For almost twenty years,

Nauerth explained, "IFOR has actively challenged the Lutheran Church to renounce" Article XVI, which has been a dubious means of legitimizing state-sanctioned violence.

Along their route, the peace pilgrims paid tribute to Anabaptist martyrs persecuted by the Lutheran Church, stopping to remember them in prayer and moments of silence. "We stand up for the right of every Christian to say 'No!' to war and 'No!' to military professions – and we no longer want to be condemned by anyone for this conviction," was the pacifist cyclists' unanimous message, a growing number of Christians agree with them. Despite this, Article XVI has never been amended or repudiated.

What's the next step? The peace pilgrims' closing statement has a suggestion: "Now it is the Lutheran Church's duty to formulate a new Article XVI, and to finally acknowledge the martyrs of the sixteenth century. . . . Christians' mission and responsibility for the world can be expressed in a better and more peaceful manner."—*Walter L. Buder*

Source: Walter L. Buder, "CA 16 – wäre besser in Wittenberg geblieben." *Vorarlberger KirchenBlatt* Nr. 38 vom 21. September 2017. Trans. Erna Albertz. Used by permission.

Memorial along with hundreds of stones dedicated to the veterans of World War I.

But the symposium was about more than remembering. As Ian Kleinsasser, one of the conference speakers, said, "Our purpose today is not to memorialize those who have endured great suffering on account of their faith, but rather to raise stones of remembrance so the principles of nonviolence and peace can be passed on to future generations." ➤
theworldwar.org/remembering-muted-voices

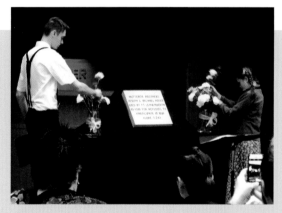

At the National World War I Museum in Kansas City, Missouri, young people representing Hutterite, *left,* and Bruderhof communities lay flowers in remembrance of men who refused to fight in World War I.

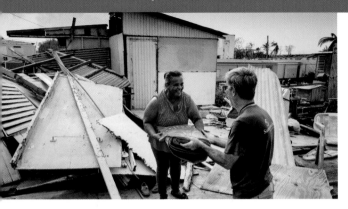

Image courtesy of Samaritan's Purse

Puerto Rico Se Levanta

Samaritan's Purse worker distributing emergency shelter kits to people in Puerto Rico

Since Hurricane Maria devastated Puerto Rico's infrastructure in September, Samaritan's Purse, a Christian relief organization, has been providing food, water, medical care, and shelter. Andreas King, a member of the Bruderhof community, volunteered with the organization for five weeks. He reports:

Ten weeks after the storm, some people still lack basic necessities like clean drinking water and tarps to cover their roofs. Despite the need, I heard only one complaint: we had brought a water purification unit to an eighty-nine-year-old blind man. "What the hell do I want with water?" he wanted to know. "Give me something real to drink!" The enthusiasm to rebuild is remarkable, and the slogan *Puerto Rico Se Levanta* – Puerto Rico Shall Rise – is everywhere, on t-shirts, flags, and cars.

As part of their long-term plan for assistance in Puerto Rico, Samaritan's Purse continues to supply generators, food, water purification units, hygiene kits, blankets, and heavy-duty plastic for shelters for families in need.

To learn more and support their work, visit *samaritanspurse.org.* ➤

Readers Respond CONTINUED . . .

(Continued from page 9)

his expense – that fills her with hope and joy in the face of a regime ready to put her in a death cell. Her hope does not rise and fall with the cycles of regimes, for her inheritance is stable and secure. She turns and looks at me, and I know the question: Where is your hope, and who is your Lord?

Jim Saladin, New York, NY

All Ploughed Up

The little congregation I am serving is deeply divided, not only politically but also in terms of how to respond and minister to gays and lesbians. I feel so incapable to be the peace-maker among them. I long for community and the *Plough* issues give me great hope and comfort, and I use excerpts as examples in my sermons. *Ruth Aukerman, Union Bridge, MD*

I received my new issue of the *Plough* today. Once again, I'm floored by its breadth and depth, and the sheer integrity of the overall undertaking. I've been struggling a lot recently with health issues and with a concomitant shakiness of faith; the *Plough* goes a long way towards reigniting that light that George Fox so famously called us all to heed.

Chris Faatz, Silverton, OR

We love reading the *Plough*. Your graphics are so wonderful, and I've often cut them out. For example, we have your design of "God's Grandeur" pasted on our mirror to have something to really look at and meditate on.

Willa Bickham,
Viva Catholic Worker House, Baltimore, MD

We welcome letters to the editor. Letters and web comments may be edited for length and clarity, and may be published in any medium. Letter should be sent with the writer's name and address to letters@plough.com. ➤

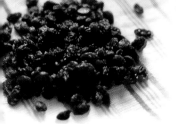

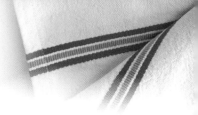

How to Homestead a Hermitage

DANA WISER

Maureen and I are on loan from the Bruderhof to Tantur Ecumenical Institute, which hosts international scholars and students on a hill outside Jerusalem. We help with Tantur's daily tasks: cooking, maintenance, olive harvesting, and library filing. When we first arrived three months ago, we had the delight of making a home out of a tiny hermitage (previously a shepherd's hut) tucked into the hill. We scrubbed down the walls in its one room, kitchen, and bath, squeezed in a collapsible table and convertible couch/bed, sewed curtains by hand, and planted flowers around the house and on the roof.

Just beyond the garden, traffic is noisy on the litter-strewn road. Joseph and Mary passed by when the traffic was donkey and camel. Stretching to the east is Shepherdsfield – yes, those shepherds' fields. Bethlehem is just down the road.

As a child, Emmy Arnold, cofounder of the Bruderhof, began anticipating each Christmas one hundred days in advance, counting down the days from September 16 in childlike expectation. Since then, Bruderhof members have made it a custom each year to dust off the carols that day and celebrate with stollen, a delicious German Christmas cake overflowing with nuts and fruit. Here in Jerusalem, we decided to celebrate One Hundred Days as a sort of Hermitage housewarming, complete with stollen and carols, together with Tantur's staff and guests. Ingredients were to hand. Almonds: knock down nuts with pole. Raisins: pick grapes, dry in sun (we have lots of both). Dried apricots: easy, Tantur serves these for breakfast. Result: the Holy Land's best stollen.

We let out the word that coffee break was at the hermitage, and staff, guests, and students – Muslims, Christians, and Jews – crowded onto our porch. Arabic coffee, bitter and aromatic, paired with sweet German stollen in a fine metaphor for peace and goodwill. In a rush of excited Arabic, our friends commended Maureen's baking and hermitage homemaking.

It was later, in the dusk, that we sang. Among the carols was "How far is it to Bethlehem?" Not very far indeed, say fifteen minutes' walk. See, there it is through the olive trees. ⤳

Shepherds' fields near Bethlehem

Dana Wiser is a member of the Bruderhof.

Image courtesy of Nabcam

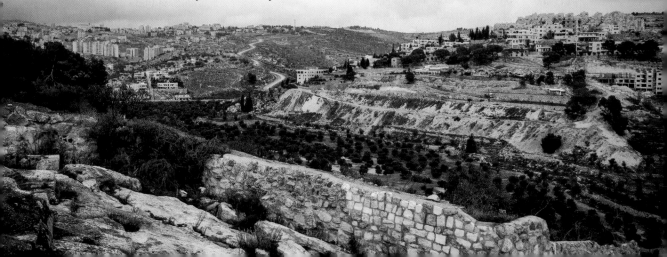

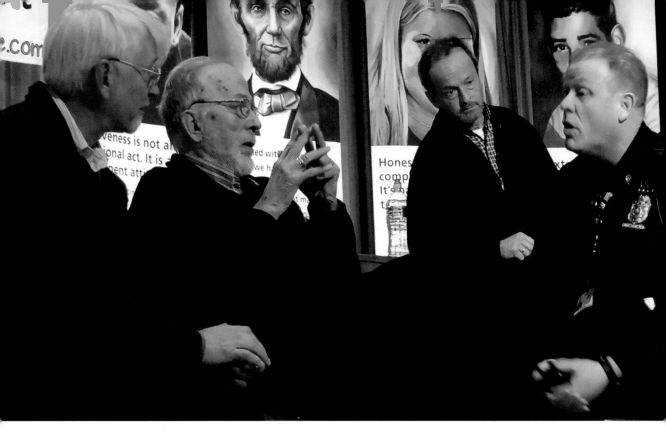

The Ministry of Reconciliation

Celebrating the Legacy of Johann Christoph Arnold

This past September, First Things editor R.R. Reno, veteran civil rights activist John M. Perkins, Professor Robert P. George, and others gathered at the Union League Club in New York City to honor the life of Johann Christoph Arnold, who died earlier this year. Arnold, who led the Bruderhof communities for two decades, was a pastor, author, and tireless worker for peace, reconciliation, and justice. The breadth of his influence was reflected in the speakers who gathered to remember him. Selections from their remarks follow.

Robert P. George

Christoph's wisdom was the fruit of a life lived in a community dedicated to Christlike simplicity and love. Those are the virtues that he modeled, not just for the members of the Bruderhof communities but for all who came into contact with him. When I was with Christoph, I never left without experiencing what it must have been like to know one of the apostles of Jesus, to know someone who had walked with Jesus, who had talked with Jesus, who had eaten with Jesus, who had confided in Jesus. That's because Christoph was, of all the people I've known in my life, the one I most think of as a friend of Jesus – a personal friend of Jesus – and Christoph lived his life as a servant of God.

Robert P. George is McCormick Professor of Jurisprudence at Princeton University.

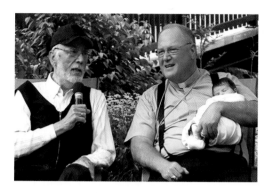

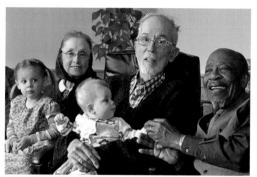

Left, with Cardinal Dolan in 2015

Right, with his wife, Verena, and John Perkins

Timothy Cardinal Dolan

I came to know Pastor Johann Christoph Arnold soon after my arrival as archbishop of New York in 2009. Here in the archdiocese we have enjoyed a deep bond with the Bruderhof. You know what the late lamented Father Benedict Groeschel once whispered to me? "They are better Catholics than I am!"

Pastor Arnold was especially courageous in his rock-solid conviction that God's word as revealed in the Bible is true and reliable and that the incarnate Word, Jesus, was the way, the truth, and the life. He was sensitive to God's presence, even in adversity and setback.

Timothy Cardinal Dolan is the Archbishop of New York.

Dr. R. R. Reno

Life in Christ, and community of the body of Christ, gives us a place to stand. Anyone visiting the Bruderhof community senses that the people in that community have a place to stand, a community of accountability, of encouragement, of teaching, of prayer, and of mutual sacrifice. As I have learned from reading Pastor Arnold and observing the Bruderhof community, this freedom is central to peace and to peacemaking, which I think is a great charism of the Bruderhof community.

R. R. Reno is editor of First Things *magazine.*

John M. Perkins

I met Christoph in the early eighties, two decades after I had gone back to Mississippi to establish what would become the Christian Community Development Association (CCDA). I was looking for a better expression of justice and love and community that reflected the New Testament. I found in Christoph another seeker for justice and righteousness. We came together to talk about how authentic reconciliation could take place in our society. So keep moving, keep seeking a greater expression of human freedom and justice.

Dr. John M. Perkins is a pastor, author, civil rights activist, and founder of CCDA.

Stacey Rein

Since 2012, the Bruderhof and the United Way of Ulster County have prevented 422 families (1,266 individuals, 67 percent of them children) from becoming homeless. The majority of these families have one thing in common: they are working. But their jobs are low wage, paying not enough to contend with life's curve balls but too much to make them eligible for government assistance. Some examples were a nurse at a local hospital whose husband left her and her three children with no child support; a single mother who was working three different jobs

Stacey Rein is president of United Way of Ulster County.

to make ends meet but became ill and needed surgery; and a family that had to provide care to a terminally ill relative. Where do families like this go? Who is going to help them? In Ulster County, we have been blessed to have the Bruderhof communities living among us; they reached out and offered assistance. As Pastor Arnold writes in his book *Cries from the Heart*: "Loving thoughts and words must be brought to fruition in concrete deeds."

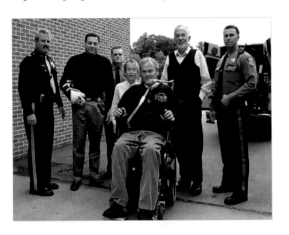

Hashim Garrett, *left,* joins Christoph signing books after a Breaking the Cycle assembly

Right, with Steven McDonald, *front*

Hashim Garrett

I would watch Christoph Arnold, with his tall, six-foot-five stature, talk to students about forgiveness in a thick German accent, and it struck me: "If he can get up in front of these kids that don't look anything like him, and with a fifty-year age gap, and talk about forgiveness, I'm gonna do it too." And I did.

I was Muslim when I met Christoph. Before our Breaking the Cycle assemblies, he would say, "Hashim, tell them that you are Muslim." And I go, *wait a minute, I'm black, I'm crippled, I used to be in a gang, and you want me to tell them I'm Muslim! Gosh, Christoph, man! Gosh! But if you say so, I'll do it, man!* And I'd go, "Look, I'm Hashim. I'm Muslim and my brother is Christian and we are here together." And he would say, "That's it! Do it." Sometimes he would go out on a ledge and talk about God in public schools. And then it would be my turn to go up and talk, and I would think, *well,*

if my brother went out on a ledge, he is not going to be out there by himself, so here it goes, yeah – "God is real." *That's right. And if you are gonna kick him out, you are gonna kick me out too.*

Hashim Garrett works with Breaking the Cycle to present programs combating school violence.

Patrick Regan

The New York State Police is an agency of five thousand sworn people. We are among the ten largest police agencies in the country. Upstate New York has many communities that are served by a local police department, a county sheriff's department, and the state police, all doing the same thing in the same area. And twenty-five years ago it was a very bad equation: a lot of parochialism and departments failing to ask for or offer assistance or share information. This was at the expense of public safety. In Ulster County, we began to meet as a police chiefs association, and in these meetings we began to break down barriers.

In 2004 I took command of the state police in Ulster and Greene counties at about the same time that Christoph and the Bruderhof's relationship with the Ulster County Police Chiefs Association really began to grow. Christoph's involvement strengthened

---

Lieutenant Colonel Patrick Regan is chief of state police in Ulster and Greene counties.

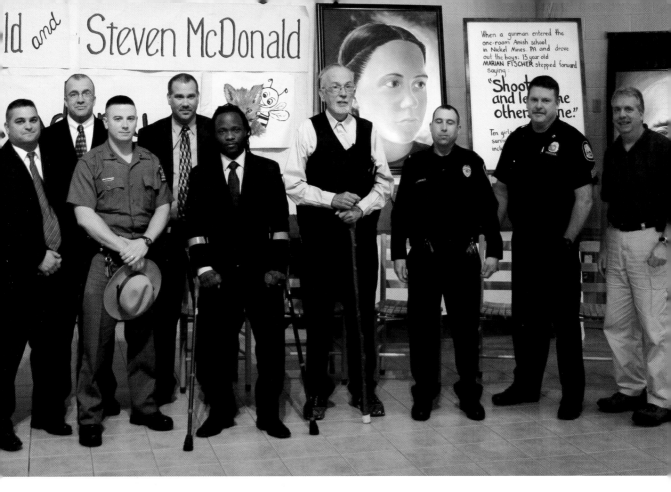

relationships within the police force through his ability to reach people on a personal level. He also forged new connections between law enforcement and the surrounding community – clergy, community groups, elected officials, and others. Personally, I was inspired by Christoph to do more outreach. You would think his message of peace and reconciliation would be at odds with law enforcement, but it really was not.

In the last years, an atmosphere of mistrust between communities and law enforcement has grown. In Ulster County there were many incidents – whether with hate groups or unfortunate encounters between law enforcement and communities – just like in communities across the country. But because of the bridges that Christoph built or inspired, there were dialogues that prevented disasters like we have seen in so many other communities.

I have also seen the impact of Christoph's counseling for law enforcement families. He was there for members of law enforcement who were traumatized by what they had seen or endured, and for families of officers who had killed themselves or been killed in the line of duty. What spoke to me about Christoph's selfless investment in these people was not so much his counseling work, but the lasting bonds that he built. Often counselors have one interaction and then it is over, but I know families who still turned to Christoph and the Bruderhof a decade after their first interaction.

Christoph's legacy is evident in the people who talk about him, who are anxious to continue his work. While he is sorely missed, he is still with us and so is his message. For that I am grateful. ➤

▶ *Watch the full event at* plough.com/arnold.

Christoph, *center,* with Hashim Garrett and other Breaking the Cycle advocates

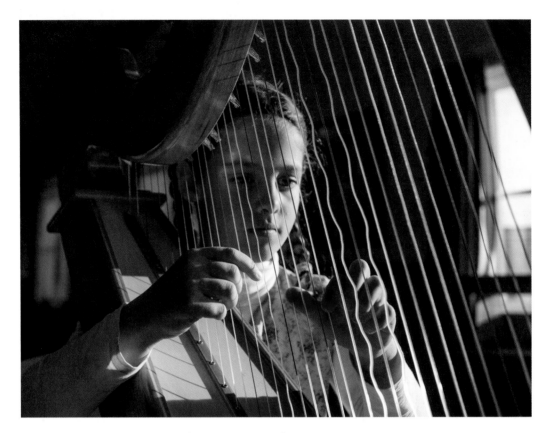

Photographs by Clare Stober

Awake the Harp

MAUREEN SWINGER

Last year, my daughter disappeared often. She'd flit through the wardrobe door to discover Mr. Tumnus, or fall down a rabbit hole to have tea with the Hatter. And she was just as unhappy at my calling her back home to help wash dishes as I had been when my own mother attempted to relocate me from Middle Earth to Later Earth because the table needed setting. Kids need a foot in both the real and the storybook worlds. But how do you strike a balance?

Balance struck all by itself last summer, when a professional harpist treated us to an impromptu outdoor concert. We were ten feet from the sound box, and as the haunting melody rippled out into the evening air, a certain daydreamer beside me woke up – and stayed awake. When the music ended, she walked through several people, never taking her eyes off those strings. The harpist was cross-examined, though she didn't seem to mind. We walked home rather dazed, and daughter informed father that she was going to play harp. He snorted in disbelief. The man can play seven instruments, but harp was not on his radar.

Maureen Swinger is an editor at Plough. *She lives at a Bruderhof in Walden, NY.*

The "you're-only-nine-think-it-over-for-a-bit" conversation went on for six months, but she kept harping on it (yes, I know).

Then some strings started to align. A friend donated a small secondhand lap harp. Another friend recommended a teacher, the harpist in the local symphony orchestra. But a lap harp gives you no room to grow, and it can't change keys. A quality lever harp, however, can cost five thousand dollars. While we were puzzling over that one, my husband and I traveled to Lancaster to staff a booth at a homeschool conference. From a distant corner of the exhibit hall, the unmistakable tones of a harp flowed over the five thousand people in attendance. We followed the sound to the booth of harp-maker Alex Marini and his family, who were playing hymns on a succession of majestic Regency harps.

We crossed paths at lunches and after-hours, and each time learned a little more, not only about harp-making, but also about the history of an instrument that has accompanied praise and prayer to God for centuries. When Alex found out that my husband is a carpenter, he told us to look into ordering blueprints and hardware for a Regency harp, for a fraction of the cost of a finished one.

What followed was the Summer of the Harp. And it must be said that the dad who had snorted at the whole concept did the lion's share of the work. But everyone helped, by scrambling around in the lumber shed for lengths of cherry wood, sanding – the three-year-old using 1000-grit sandpaper, so it didn't matter how much energy was expended – gluing, painting, and staining. Oh, and tuning! It took fifty tune-ups before the strings held their pitch faithfully enough to add the key levers. Now the first Christmas songs are echoing through our house: "In the

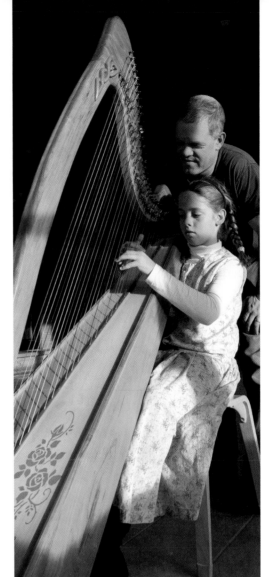

After three months of building, father and daughter enjoy the first notes.

"Shout for joy to the Lord, all the earth, burst into jubilant song with music; make music to the Lord with the harp, with the harp and the sound of singing."
Psalm 98

bleak midwinter," "Oh Holy Night. . . ." There is nothing in the world like the sound of a harp. Is there a downside? Maybe. Now dad and daughter squabble over who gets to play . . . and neither of them will do the dishes. ✎

▶ *Watch the harp-building process and hear the debut performance at* bruderhof.com/harp.

The

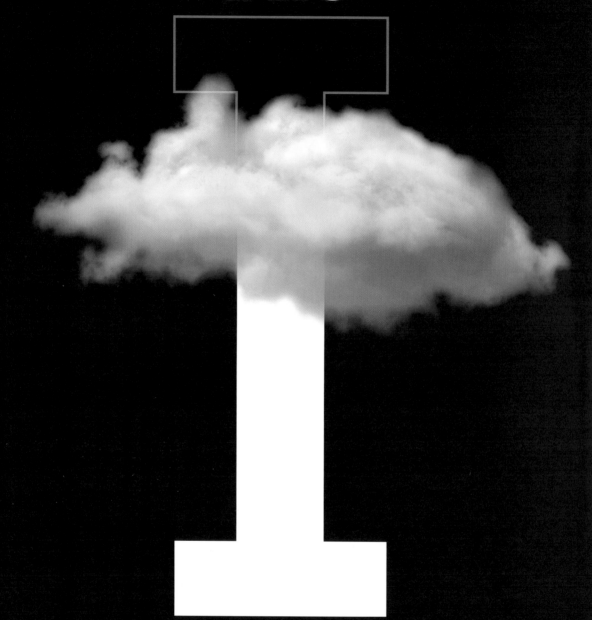

mmortality
machine

Transhumanism
and the race to beat death

MICHAEL PLATO

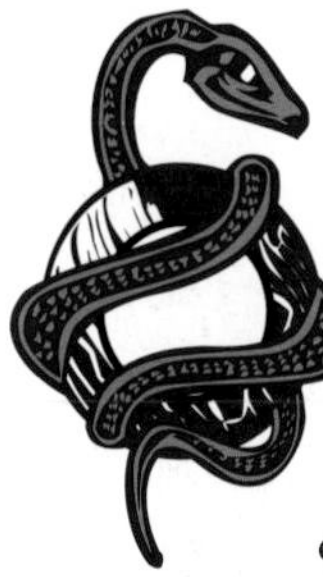

O f the many ideologies and isms to emerge in recent years, transhumanism, which promotes striving for immortality through technology, has to be one of the quirkiest. But its advocates are dead serious. Silicon Valley tech magnates Peter Thiel, Larry Ellison, Sergey Brin, Larry Page, and Bill Maris have already poured hundreds of millions of dollars into research dedicated to slowing or even stopping the aging process. And the Transhumanist Party's presidential candidate, Zoltan Istvan, who recently criss-crossed the nation in a coffin-shaped RV called the Immortality Bus, claims that death itself can be eradicated in "eight to twelve years, with enough funding."

Beyond Silicon Valley, transhumanism is extending its reach into intellectual and spiritual realms. Though still largely rejected by the mainstream academy, transhumanism has found support in surprising places, for example at Oxford University's Future of Humanity Institute. Transhumanism's movers and shakers, made up predominantly of tech entrepreneurs and independent "visionaries," have held conferences, published widely, and funded research, much of it via a think tank called Humanity Plus.

The transhumanist movement seeks to improve human intelligence, physical strength, and the five senses by technological means. Transhumanists are often also interested in the idea of "technological singularity," a hypothesized moment in the development of computing power when a true artificial intelligence emerges. This would, its adherents believe, spark an explosion of technological growth, leading to unimaginable, but positive, changes in human society. In certain versions of this scenario, humans and computers would merge, and humanity as a whole would be brought to a new stage of development that would transcend biology.

Above all, transhumanists seek to extend life, even to the point of eliminating death

Michael John Plato is assistant professor of intellectual history and Christian thought at Colorado Christian University.

Image from iStock/ xochicalco

altogether. This latter possibility has led to the emergence of one of transhumanism's strangest fads: cryopreservation facilities. These businesses will, for a price, freeze the bodies (or heads) of those who believe that technological resurrection will be possible someday, that a cure for a fatal disease will be discovered, or that it will be possible to upload one's mind into a computer, or even into a new body. It is this aspect of transhumanism that most closely links it to religious faith.

Is transhumanism fundamentally incompatible with Christian faith? Already there are "Christian Transhumanists," who have their own association, complete with website and conferences. The term, they note, has roots in Christian thought: it originates with Dante and appears in the work of Pierre Teilhard de Chardin. According to the Christian Transhumanist Association, "the intentional use of technology, coupled with following Christ, will empower us to become more human." But what if the goal is now clearly to become *more than human?* As such, transhumanism has had a particularly strong appeal to Mormons. The Mormon Transhumanist Association, while not officially endorsed by the LDS Church, meets regularly in Salt Lake City, and seeks to link aspects of Mormon theology, such as the doctrine that states that humans will evolve into gods, to transhumanist goals, particularly self-attained immortality.

Transhumanism has not been without its articulate detractors. Rosi Braidotti, a prominent leftist European philosopher, dismisses transhumanism as having "contempt for the flesh" and being a "fantasy of escape from the finite materiality of the enfleshed self." Neoconservative political scientist Francis Fukuyama calls transhumanism "the most dangerous idea in the world." In his book *Our Posthuman Future: Consequences of the*

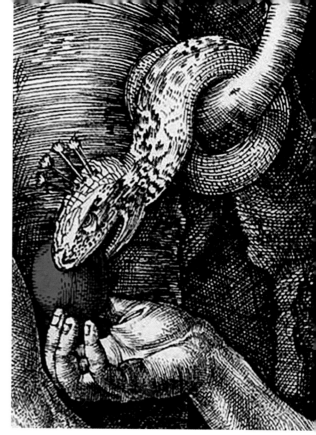

Biotechnology Revolution, he argues that all the technological means of self-advancement proposed by transhumanism would "come at a frightful moral cost" and lead to a nightmarish dystopian future.

To believe that some of the proposed technologies are even possible takes no small leap of faith. As journalist Anna Wiener recently noted in the *New Republic,* transhumanism may be based more on wishful thinking than realistic expectations of technological development. She notes, regarding cryonic freezing, that "to date, science has not suggested that reanimation will ever be possible." The dream of uploading one's mind to a computer, or to a new body, she writes, "remains just that: a dream." Mark O'Connell, in *To Be a Machine: Adventures Among Cyborgs, Utopians, Hackers, and the Futurists Solving the Modest Problem of Death,* argues that while transhumanists have begun to pop up around the world, the idea is still very much a child of California culture, linked as it is to that state's history of self-improvement fads and crazes rather than to substantial scientific developments.

Over the last few years a number of science fiction films have explored transhumanist ideas and expectations. Johnny Depp appeared in *Transcendence* (2014) as a scientist whose mind is uploaded into a computer system, while *Ghost in the Shell* (2017), starring Scarlett Johansson, imagined a world where human brains could be transferred to superior robot bodies. The Justin Timberlake vehicle *In Time* (2011) forecast a future in which technology allows people to remain young and beautiful for decades or even centuries. *In Time* points out another aspect of this transhumanist dream often missing from the narrative of its real-world advocates: namely, that if such technology becomes possible, it would likely be available only to the superrich. It's a point that Christine Emba raised in a 2016 piece for the *Washington Post*: the benefits of transhumanism will, she warns, "accrue only to the upper classes," and "inequality will be entrenched in ways deeper than just wealth, fundamentally challenging our egalitarian ideals."

Yet advocates insist that the technologies of transhumanism, whatever they may be, would merely be extensions of assistive technologies we already have. After all, what are eyeglasses, pacemakers, organ transplants, and artificial limbs? These technologies enhance and even extend life. And while the rich may have first dibs, as these technologies develop they become accessible to the middle and lower class, as has been the case with other techno-logical developments.

Despite its flavor of billionaire self-empowerment, New Age enthusiasm, and science fiction fantasy, transhumanism nevertheless addresses a fundamental hope that Christians can affirm: death is an enemy that must someday be defeated and ultimately transcended. The apostle Paul writes, "[Christ] must reign until he has put all his enemies under his feet. The last enemy to be destroyed is death" (1 Cor. 15: 25–26). That so many atheist transhumanists look at death with hostility and hunger for immortality should be, at a very basic level, encouraging for Christians.

After all, Christians believe death has already been defeated in the death and bodily resurrection of Jesus Christ. Because of what God has done in Christ, Christians are never without hope of their own future resurrection. For many transhumanists, this business of awaiting future glory may seem pallid, but by comparison, how much more feeble is it to await a desperately hoped-for awakening from cryo-freeze?

> "By trying to be like God, we reject our dependence on God as our creator, choosing instead to try to live as though we are our own creators."

That Christians place their ultimate hope in Christ's final victory over death does not mean they can't fight against things that threaten life and happiness here and now. They ought to welcome technologies that result in improved human wellness – those eyeglasses, pacemakers, artificial limbs, and organ transplants – as long as these technologies are restorative. Even if these technologies happen to enhance our natural abilities (for example, people with artificial legs are winning races), such technologies are still in accord with our human nature; they do not seek to transform us into something else entirely.

Transhumanism sharply diverges from Christianity in its rejection of the idea that our human bodies are good as is because they are created by a good God. That Christ himself has a human body and possesses a human nature affirms the goodness and completeness of the human. In this, transhumanism is more akin to the Gnosticism of centuries past, which treated the body as malleable or even outright repugnant and disposable. Transhumanism is likewise connected with other movements of our time, such as transgenderism, which rejects the idea that gender is given by God and not ours to choose.

Christians believe that humanity was created in the image of God. That image, while not understood physically, is not autonomous and self-determined but is utterly dependent upon the God whom it reflects. This is what Dietrich Bonhoeffer means when he distinguishes between seeking to live as an image of God on the one hand, and giving in to the serpent's temptation to seek "to be like God" on the other. By trying "to be like God," we reject our dependence on God as our creator, choosing instead to try to live as though we are our own creators.

For the transhumanist, overcoming humanity's limitations is fundamentally grounded in the values of individual freedom and choice. Death is just another unacceptable limitation on human freedom. Theologian Brent Waters puts it bluntly when he states that, for the transhumanist, "it is only when mortality has been vanquished that we can be truly free." In its self-centered search for infinite autonomy and freedom, transhumanism promises an immortality that is a grotesque mimicry of God-given immortality. It hijacks the Christian promise of life everlasting. Immortality becomes a commodity, one that each person seeks for himself. A vision of this godless immortality and its banality and emptiness can be found in Jorge Luis Borges's short story "The Immortal":

> There is nothing very remarkable about being immortal; with the exception of mankind, all creatures are immortal, for they know nothing of death. What is divine, terrible, and incomprehensible is to *know* oneself immortal.

It is indeed a horrific prospect to be left trapped in our own unredeemed selves for eternity. There is a word, after all, for such an eternity: we call it hell. Merely extending our lives is not the kind of immortality we are yearning for. The Christians' hope, instead, is in eternal life as a result of entrance into the kingdom of God. Yes, we expect a real, physical resurrection, but it is a resurrection that comes as an undeserved gift of a loving God. That is a promise that no technology could even pretend to try to keep. ⤙

Image from iStock / sorbetto

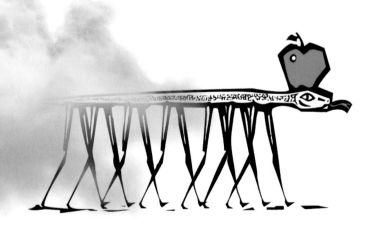

The Immortality Delusion

A Reading from C. S. Lewis

What's really at stake in the push for trans-humanism? Writing in 1945, C. S. Lewis presciently addressed this question in his novel That Hideous Strength. *Here, at a meeting in a secretive research compound known as the National Institute of Coordinated Experiments, the scientist Filostrato is confiding to the new-comer Mark what the Institute's goals really are:*

"In us organic life has produced Mind. It has done its work. After that we want no more of it. We do not want the world any longer furred over with organic life, like what you call the blue mould – all sprouting and budding and breeding and decaying. We must get rid of it. By little and little, of course. Slowly we learn how. Learn to make our brains live with less and less body: learn to build our bodies directly with chemicals, no longer have to stuff them full of dead brutes and weeds. Learn how to reproduce ourselves without copulation. . . .

"The world I look forward to is the world of perfect purity. The clean mind and the clean minerals. What are the things that most offend the dignity of man? Birth and breeding and death. How if we are about to discover that man can live without any of the three? . . .

"For the moment, I speak only to inspire you. I speak that you may know what can be done: what shall be done here. This Institute – *Dio mio,* it is for something better than housing and vaccinations and faster trains and curing the people of cancer. It is for the conquest of death: or for the conquest of organic life, if you prefer. They are the same thing. It is to bring out of that cocoon of organic life which sheltered the babyhood of mind the New Man, the man who will not die, the artificial man, free from Nature. Nature is the ladder we have climbed up by, now we kick her away. . . .

> "Nature is the ladder we have climbed up by. Now we kick her away."

"Of course . . . the power will be confined to a number – a small number – of individual men. Those who are selected for eternal life."

"And you mean," said Mark, "it will then be extended to all men?"

"No," said Filostrato. "I mean it will then be reduced to one man. You are not a fool, are you, my young friend? All that talk about the power of Man over Nature – Man in the abstract – is only for the *canaglia.* You know as well as I do that Man's power over Nature means the power of some men over other men with Nature as the instrument. There is no such thing as Man – it is a word. There are only men. No! It is not Man who will be omnipotent, it is some one man, some immortal man. . . . It may be you. It may be me."

Source: C. S. Lewis, *That Hideous Strength* (Scribner, 1996). Used with permission.

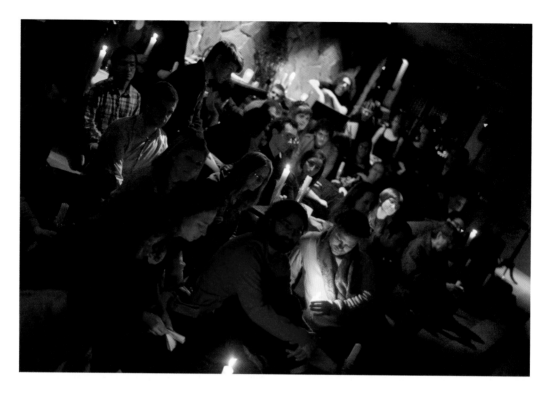

Simulating Religion

A Christian takes stock of Silicon Valley's rationalist community

ALEXI SARGEANT

Bay Area rationalists at a Secular Solstice celebration

Christians, by and large, don't like tech culture. To many, Silicon Valley seems irredeemably hostile to New Testament values. The young people working there, in this view, are hedonistic digital yuppies riding a fiscally conservative, socially liberal ideology to its dystopian endpoint, atomized individuals with no ties of loyalty except to over-powerful and under-regulated tech firms.

There are good reasons for this skepticism, but it's missing something. Strange and surprising subcultures are thriving in the hothouse of tech country. Among them is a loose-knit community calling themselves "rationalists." Based in California, this group is united by a heady mix of futuristic idealism and communitarianism.

As an outsider, I'm by turns fascinated and frightened by the rationalists and their worldview. They can be articulate critics of the tech world's dominant ideology. They're also social experimenters who serve as their own guinea pigs.

I first came across the rationalist community by clicking links on the blog of the woman I would one day marry, Leah Libresco. My wife thinks her conversion to Catholicism is partly attributable to discussions she was having on the rationalist internet. Leah loved

---

Alexi Sargeant is a theater director and culture critic who writes from New York City.

the rationalists' focus on seeking truth above all else and investigating ways to set aside bias in order to do that. Leah says, "I was particularly taken with an essay by the Bay Area thinker Eliezer Yudkowsky on the virtues of rationality, especially that of *lightness* – holding oneself so as to be ready to be moved by evidence. It helped me, as Christianity became more and more plausible, to be ready to give in – to let myself be moved by truth, and ultimately, by God."

While I don't know of many other rationalists who've made a similar journey, Leah's experience has shown me that Christians need to take the rationalists' ideals seriously. We can affirm their commitment to learning and living the truth; we can applaud their attempts to create community; and we can take a cue from their desire to do good on a global scale. We can also learn from their hunger for the sacred, a desire for meaning that drives them to engineer new secular sacraments and that offers a vivid glimpse into a different kind of religious seeking.

Origins

The rationalist community formed on the internet, first on the economics blog *Overcoming Bias* and then, especially, on its spinoff website, LessWrong. This site was cofounded by Eliezer Yudkowsky, a self-taught researcher in the world of artificial intelligence (AI) frightened by the possibility that these programs might one day become unfriendly to humankind and frustrated that people in his field did not prioritize investigating safety measures to protect humanity from them. What if we created something much smarter and therefore more powerful than us and it didn't share our

> **I'm by turns fascinated and frightened by rationalists and their world view.**

values but instead sought an alien goal of its own – like repurposing all the matter in the universe into paper clips?

Yudkowsky felt he could best encourage AI safety research by creating a culture of rational thinking. LessWrong is an attempt at creating that culture, and it has attracted a crowd interested in AI safety. The community has also come to discuss and sometimes emulate Yudkowsky's other interests: the Bayesian theory of statistics, polyamory, and a sci-fi future of cryonic freezing and mind-uploading immortality.

Rationalists take a somewhat paradoxical approach to keeping hold of their humanity in the face of technology. Apprehensive of the potential anti-human power of artificial intelligence, some in the community ponder the possibility that humanity might have to be changed radically to defeat death, perhaps shedding this mortal coil to become digital beings. By undergoing this change, we will preserve what they see as those things that are crucial to our humanity, like our boundless curiosity and creativity. (Our physical selves are, for the vast majority in the community, not intrinsic to who we are.) One rationalist, Alex Altair, says he believes that not only could we someday live indefinitely, but we could alter our minds so as to always be learning new things and "trying on different personalities."

Altair, a software developer, was first drawn into the community by Yudkowsky's fan-fiction epic *Harry Potter and the Methods of Rationality*. He loves the rationalists' "world-scale ambition" and lack of bias toward localness, either in time or space. "Why care only about Earth when there are so many planets out there?" He sees no reason not to

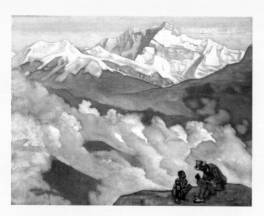

Finding Someone to Worship

CHRISTOPH F. BLUMHARDT

Nicholas
Roerich,
*Pearl of
Searching*

Have you ever looked at the world to see what is driving it, what it has dreamed up in the way of worshiping God in some way? The whole creation is thirsting for God. Human history is but a burning thirst for God. "What do I care about God!" people say, and yet they go on to create their own gods anyway. And then they cry out for God's mercy as soon as life overwhelms them.

Whether people are pagan, Muslim, or Christian, or find it impossible to believe, Jesus hears their cries. So suffer with those you meet, and love them. All the misery of this world stems from a deep thirst that results from living far away from God. The heavy load of sin that presses down on people with such satanic power leads millions into wrong and perverse ways, into dark paths of idolatry and sin, confusion and twisted thoughts about God. All the more, keep your heart open to hear their heartache. ➤

Christoph Friedrich Blumhardt (1842–1919) was a German pastor and religious socialist who influenced theologians such as Dietrich Bonhoeffer, Eberhard Arnold, Emil Brunner, and Karl Barth with his unconventional ideas about faith and the kingdom of God.

Source: *Everyone Belongs to God* (Plough, 2015) pp. 84–85.

take the whole world – indeed, the whole of time – as a playing field. After all, if humanity survives to colonize the universe, he posits, it is likely that the vast majority of people who will ever exist are in our future. Averting existential risk and helping those future people is a major goal, a value that he holds because, he says, "All humans are pretty similar, compared to other objects in the universe."

Altair thinks that anyone who reasons with enough "hardiness of mind" will come to see AI as one of the most important risks we face as a species. Though he admits his apocalyptic worries can sound absurd, Altair thinks they are gaining steam among people who think seriously about these things, starting with Nick Bostrom (author of *Superintelligence: Paths, Dangers, Strategies*) and spreading to Bill Gates and Elon Musk.

Rationalist Rituals

Despite their commitment to the idea that genuine community can exist on the internet, many rationalists have affirmed the importance of community in the flesh as well. Bay Area rationalists have even congregated in group houses. Another physical gathering place is the Center for Applied Rationality (CFAR), which advances the cause of combating existential AI risk by running intensive four-day workshops on rationality. The 2016 annual LessWrong survey of rationalists had about three thousand respondents, perhaps a ballpark number for the community's size.

In building a shared culture, some rationalists draw on the example of religious communities. In a recent post on his blog *Compass Rose*, Ben Hoffman weighs the pros and cons of becoming a Quaker, given their track record of coming to what he considers correct positions (like abolitionism and pacifism) before the rest of society. In another post,

Image from WikiArt (public domain)

he advocates the wisdom of Jewish Sabbath restrictions as a sanity check on the modern world: "If something like the Orthodox Sabbath seems impossibly hard, or if you try to keep it but end up breaking it every week – as my Reform Jewish family did – then you should consider that perhaps, despite the propaganda of the palliatives [e.g., fast food, Facebook], *you are in a permanent state of emergency*." Contemporary society drowns us in noisy demands, he argues, producing spread-too-thin communities and lonely individuals.

Christians need to take the rationalists' ideals seriously.

Altair has attended and helped organize iterations of the rationalists' Secular Solstice celebration. The event had its genesis in rationalists' observations of other cultures' various rituals and traditions. "It may be weird to engineer that, but we're all engineers," says Altair. The first Secular Solstice event was spearheaded by musician Raymond Arnold in 2013. Arnold wrote in an introduction to a book of Solstice songs: "I have some oddly specific, nuanced, and weird beliefs. And I had the hubris to arrange a night of carefully designed ritual for myself and my friends to celebrate them." The Solstice's central structure is based on light and darkness. Attendees bring and light "oil lamps, LEDs, plasma balls and imitation lightsabers" that are eventually extinguished so that participants can experience darkness together. Finally, everything is lit again, a symbol of a brighter future. It's a powerful visual, one that feels like a processed and repurposed Easter vigil, though it was apparently conceived in design as "reverse Hanukkah."

Music is a central component of the event. One of Altair's favorites is the curiously titled "The Word of God," a deist encomium to scientific investigation with a refrain of variations on "Humans wrote the Bible, God wrote the rocks." After a few Solstices, Arnold amped up the song's secularism by altering the lyrics to "Humans wrote the book of earth, time wrote the rocks" and variations thereon – God and the Bible have disappeared even as objects of deist critique.

Apart from songs, the event features secular sermons and mindfulness exercises. Many of these focus on hopes and fears for the far-flung future, asking the attendees, "Are we being good ancestors?" It struck me that although Christians' vision of the future is different, this would be a useful question to ask ourselves as well.

The Secular Solstice event spread to seven cities by 2016, and attendance has steadily increased, with people coming for the music, speeches, and communal solidarity on offer. Altair sees the celebration as hugely successful at capturing the trust-building and bonding functions of religious rituals.

Rationalist Religion?

There's a parallel between the rationalists' efforts to engineer ritual profundity and their way of describing human beings' interior life. Rob Bensinger, research communications manager at Machine Intelligence Research Institute (MIRI), told me, "We can think of human minds as a kind of computer, or (if we reserve the word 'computer' for engineered artifacts) as a naturally occurring system that a computer could emulate." Altair was confident that human minds could eventually be simulated perfectly: "The physical process that makes up the mind is all there is to the mind. If you simulate that in some other medium, you get the same thing." David Souther, a CFAR alumnus and software engineer who

The Rationalsphere

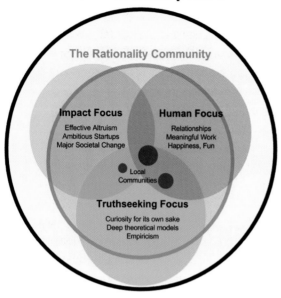

The Rationality Community

Impact Focus
Effective Altruism
Ambitious Startups
Major Societal Change

Human Focus
Relationships
Meaningful Work
Happiness, Fun

Local Communities

Truthseeking Focus
Curiosity for its own sake
Deep theoretical models
Empiricism

A graph from the LessWrong website showing "what people [in the rationalist community] care about"

considers himself on the periphery of the rationalist community, made the comparison more bluntly: "What makes us different from computers? Today, efficiency of processing." He assured me that we'll see computers as efficient as human minds in, at most, a few decades, and machine consciousness will probably follow that.

As with minds, so with holidays. If no phenomenon, not even human consciousness, is more or other than its underlying physical process, then simulating the relevant parts of the process in a new medium will also produce that phenomenon. Take candlelight, closeness, and song; run the simulation with rationalists; and – *ta-da!* – the output is culture. Altair was intrigued by the analogy that the rationalist community was a sort of simulation of a religious community. "Reductionism is one of our primary tools that we tend to reach for first," he said.

This suggestive parallel, however, doesn't mean rationalists are religious believers. To the contrary: LessWrong's 2016 survey shows that believers in God were a tiny minority, with only 3.7 percent of respondents identifying as "committed theists" – a distant fourth after "atheist and not spiritual" (the winner by a mile at 48 percent), "agnostic" (8 percent), and "atheist but spiritual" (5.5 percent). Despite this, the problems the rationalists are trying to solve are essentially theological: What would a just, omnipotent entity be like? What eternal future should humans desire, and how can we get there? Thus the religious casts the rationalists take on, from Solstices to Sabbath-envy, shouldn't be so surprising. The question from the AI research branch of the rationalists is "How can we responsibly make a god?" And the answer from the community-building branch is "First, make a church."

Altair, Arnold, and others are responding to a lacuna in the present world not by shrugging but by trying to build something to fill it. After all, rationalists like Hoffman are quite right that mainstream contemporary culture is in many ways inhumane, even dehumanizing. Christians have even more resources to draw on to make this critique and to model our lives on. I wish more of us were as willing as the rationalists to look foolish in the eyes of the dominant culture in service of wholeness (and in our case, holiness).

To act more effectively on these good desires for wholeness, rationalists could use a more robust anthropology. The reductionism to which the rationalists so often resort poses challenges for a group that is seeking to preserve humanity against the threat of its potential extinction. What, in the minds of the rationalist community, are these humans whose well-being they are eager to promote? One thing that frustrated me in my conversation with Altair was the way he treated each person's values as almost immutable, the way he resisted making normative claims about what we *should* value. Surely, rationality shouldn't only help us achieve whatever we happen to want; shouldn't it also help us shape our desires in accord with truth? According to Altair, this is a contentious issue among rationalists, though he himself has "cheated" by simply making his fundamental goal knowing true things. Though I tried, I could not get him to concede that some of those truths might be moral facts about human purpose.

Sexual morality, for example, is an area in which rationalists' views clash starkly with what Christianity teaches as true. It's almost as though rationalists view monogamous marriage as something like an outdated technology. Some Bay Area rationalists have paired off in unconventional ways such as handfasting, a novel commitment ceremony that binds the participating couple for a year and a day. In LessWrong's 2016 survey, 13 percent of respondents said they preferred polyamorous relationships. In my view, here the rationalists are blind to grave dangers: they are making themselves – and, increasingly, their children – human test subjects in a social experiment that is bound to prove destructive.

The LessWrong rationalists have their critics. RationalWiki, another rationalist group, heaps the same scorn on Yudkowsky as it does on creationists and UFO conspiracy theorists, and essentially accuses him of leading a personality cult. But LessWrong participants are not blind to these dangers and write long sequences of blog posts on spotting and correcting bad aspects of cults. Rob Bensinger (MIRI) says he responds to this critique of the LessWrong community by

asking the critic to be more specific: "I think 'culty' can be gesturing at a lot of different things, some of which are really important to be wary of in small 'idea-oriented' communities (the tendencies toward conformism and overconfidence), and others of which aren't inherently concerning (such as weirdness)."

The Yudkosky-as-cult-leader charge is undercut by the fact that plenty of rationalists are willing to critique him. When his utilitarianism leads him to abhorrent positions such as claiming it would be right to torture an innocent person if it saved a sufficiently high number of future people from minor annoyances, other rationalists in his community make counterarguments. More light-heartedly, a humor page on LessWrong collected Chuck Norris–style Yudkowsky facts like "There was no ice age. Eliezer Yudkowsky just persuaded the planet to sign up for cryonics."

Another stick commonly used to beat the rationalists is the infamous episode of Roko's Basilisk, a 2010 thought experiment. A LessWrong contributor posited that a future, *friendly,* omnipotent AI might be obligated to recreate and then torture a simulation of anyone who didn't do enough to bring about its existence. As each day we aren't ruled by a benevolent god-computer is a needless waste of human life, the future AI might need to institute these punishments in order to motivate us to contribute all we can to AI research. (Yes, this does involve all sorts of mental time travel, but that's a detail; don't forget rationalists like to think globally in time and space.) The thought experiment's force depends on the utilitarianism common to the community: an action is right if it leads to the

> ## The events focus on hopes and fears for the future, asking, "Are we being good ancestors?"

greatest happiness for the greatest number of people. And it was, for some of those in the community, remarkably upsetting.

Yudkowsky deleted the original post and banned discussion of it, citing the psychological harm it could cause readers who agonized over it. The whole incident is commonly used as evidence that the rationalists are crazy. But, at least in the 2016 LessWrong survey, only 10 percent of rationalists reported ever feeling any sort of anxiety about Roko's Basilisk, and vanishingly few were still worrying about it. All in all, the episode mostly proves that some rationalists took seriously the stated eternal-life-or-eternal-death stakes of their beliefs. If hell does not exist, it might be necessary to invent it.

The Shape of Alief

In the end, I find I can only describe rationalists by using a term they introduced me to: *alief,* which means one of those attitudes that lie below our articulated beliefs but still inform our actions. Rationalists may not believe a spiritual creed, but many seem to share a strong alief in reverence, communion, and liturgy – even in the power of their pseudo-sacraments to help humanity pull itself out of the darkness and reach eternal life among the stars. I believe their desires – for meaning, for solidarity, for immortality – are true, truer even than they themselves know, even though they believe these things must be created by man in the face of an uncaring universe, not received as graces from the Creator.

On this front, Christians can engage those involved in the rationalist project. These atheists don't live in a "disenchanted" world, but in one where their actions and beliefs

have meaning, even eschatological meaning. The shape of their secular hope, the desire for a future ruled by a benevolent intelligence, points towards the inescapable human longing for the kingdom of God. Of course, in their enthusiastic pursuit of truth, community, and techno-futurist salvation, they have invented some novel errors. Yet, these are people with whom we can and should be talking, though it might require learning their idiosyncratic language. And, fortunately, one of their virtues is an openness to talking to people radically at odds with them.

> **Rationalists are people with whom we can and should be talking.**

I told my rationalist interlocutors that, frankly, I feared the rationalist community could come to represent the social equivalent of the unfriendly AI that Yudkowsky is worried about. After all, what he fears is the rule of a superintelligent moral naïf. The rationalists are a new, smart, powerful entity, not particularly bound by conventional morality, interested in rebuilding the world in their image. How can we be sure they aren't turning themselves and us into paper clips – maximizing an idiosyncratic goal at the expense of normal human values?

Altair said he thought many rationalists would take the comparison as a compliment, since it means I view them as very smart. But he also said he could understand someone fearing the scale of rationalist aims: "World-scale ambition comes with a world-scale potential for failure – not failure, destruction." However, Altair asks critics of rationalism to talk to the rationalist community, so together we can test our beliefs and improve our mental map of the world. He says our common destiny should motivate cooperation: "Help us figure out how to make this one future that we share a good one." ⤳

The Soul of Work

EBERHARD ARNOLD

THE ONLY WORK a person can do with his or her whole soul comes from love. And there is no love that does not get to work. Love is work, work of muscle and mind, heart and soul. This kingdom of love, therefore, this kingdom of the church and of the coming rule of God, must be a kingdom of work. Work – truly unselfish work – animated by the spirit of brotherhood will be the mark of the future, the character of the humankind to be. Where all our senses are consecrated and all our tools dedicated; where everything physical becomes holy and all activity in manual work a joy; where there is zest, the bubbling vigor of enthusiasm in work, there is the kingdom of the future!

Humans have been appointed to rule this earth, to move the earth with their tools and shape matter for this work. But brutal degradation clings like a blight, a curse, to the tools, the factories, the machines, and the industry of today. People are forced to perform soulless labor for which they have no heart or quickening of spirit, and in which no community results.

We cannot yet tell in detail how this communal love of work with its voluntary nature and joy in creativity will become practical reality. We do not know to what extent mechanized industry will be struck when the works of the devil are destroyed. The evolution of work has arrived at a deadlock: division of labor and victimization of people. Love must also become inventive in the technical area, so that soul, oversight, and unity are brought into every piece of work once more.

To put effort into one's work, exerting one's powers, is a good thing even if it makes one sweat. But breathing chemicals, swallowing coal dust, getting lead poisoning, and becoming mentally stultified is an infernal murder, one which we must abolish if we are to become truly human. When

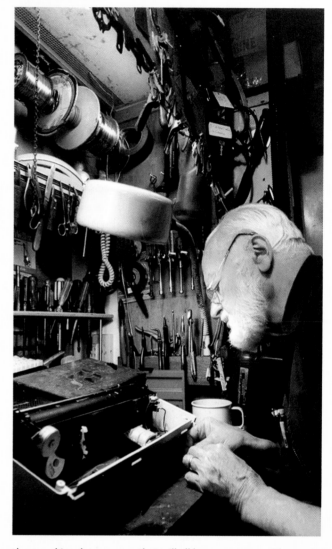

the new kingdom comes, that will all be overcome and done away with.

This is not some fantastic, unattainable future; on the contrary, it is the quiet reality of a church already emerging today. God *is* – everywhere and always. We cannot make the kingdom of God – that is impossible – but we can live in God's kingdom all the time. Christ comes to us. And as certainly as this is true for individuals, personally, it will be fulfilled as a fact in world history. ⇒

The repair man and his tools: Arnold Mommsen, a Bruderhof member, salvages a typewriter.

Eberhard Arnold (1883–1935) was the founding editor of Plough.

Source: "Community and the Future of Work," unpublished manuscript, 1921, trans. Emmy Barth Maendel (Bruderhof Historical Archive, EA 20/21a).

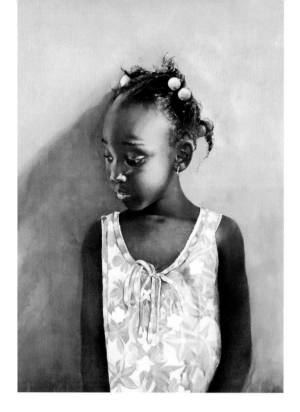

Why Children Need

White Space

JOHANN CHRISTOPH ARNOLD

Stephen
Scott Young,
Little Cindy

hildren of the twenty-first century can navigate distant worlds from their video game controllers, but are often not equipped with an understanding of the real world outside the window. Fascinating entertainment options have them hooked almost as soon as they can focus their eyes. As parents and teachers, we know that too much technology is bad for children. And we've all heard horror stories about cyberbullying, easily accessible porn sites, and online sexual predators. Parents can try to put controls on what their children can see and limit their access time. But what if the technology itself turns out to be bad for childhood?

Rhonda Gillespie is an infant and toddler specialist who has worked in early childhood education for decades. When I asked her what she thought about technology and children, she shared her own story:

Johann Christoph Arnold (1940–2017) was an author and senior pastor of the Bruderhof communities.

"I have seen a devastating impact on children over the last twenty years. Technology attacks the foundation necessary for healthy development. When I was a child, our neighborhood was safe and I played outside every day with my friends. We used our creativity and imagination, enhanced our problem solving skills, and developed healthy bodies. But by the time my son was growing up, I rarely saw neighborhood children playing outside. The trend had shifted, and the outdoors was perceived to be unsafe.

"I had to return to work full time, which meant long days and less evening time to play and enjoy the outdoors with my son. The biggest mistake I made was purchasing him his first video game console. It started off with rules and time limits, but as time progressed, so did the hours at the game controller.

"At the beginning, it seemed like a win-win: he was interacting with children from all over the world and could casually socialize with his age group. He became good at some games and his confidence rose. I always thought that at some point he would find friends to play with in the neighborhood. Socialization has always been a challenge for him, and video game companies often bill their products as a bridge to forming connections. Now I feel he was denied the chance to develop healthy interactions.

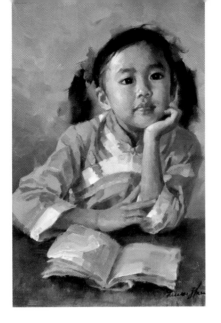

Just as books require white space, so do children.

"My son is seventeen years old now. He will text all day long. He says he is comfortable talking to people on the computer because he does not get bullied. But the flip side is that he did not learn to work through those awkward childhood moments that are an opportunity for growth. If he had never had the choice of online 'friends,' would he have learned better social skills?"

Jie Wei Zhou,
Study Girl

We know that physical health is affected by screen time – especially eyesight, hearing, and weight. But we also need to consider how it attacks a child's soul. Many children find themselves unable to communicate with a real person who requires a thoughtful verbal response. More and more young children arrive at preschool with speech difficulties; some do not speak at all. Since this is a diagnosable trait in the autism spectrum, how many children may be categorized as autistic when they have simply not had the opportunity to learn human interaction?

In my conflict resolution work in schools, I sometimes speak with teens who don't know who they are – what is real about themselves and what is a mask. They have spent their growing years using several different personas or avatars in various imaginary worlds, and if they can make these false fronts more

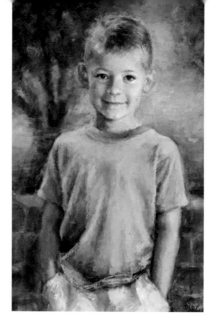

glamorous and bold than any mere human can hope to be, we should not be surprised that they come to hate themselves. This leads to desperation, depression, and in all too many cases, suicide.

There is no easy way to relieve the burden that technology places on children. But if we love them, we can't slip into resignation just because we don't know where to start. One way to take action is to give children more "white space." In a book, white space is the room between the lines of type, the margins, the extra space at the beginning of a chapter. It allows the type to "breathe" and gives the eye a place to rest. White space is not something you're conscious of when you read a book. It is what isn't there. But if it were gone, you'd notice it right away. It is the key to a well-designed page.

Just as books require white space, so do children. They need room to grow, in a space shielded from the onslaught of the information age. It does not take a brilliant mind to see the effects of a lack of white space. When children are overwhelmed by entertainment, material goods, high-pressure academics, and frequently unstable home life, it's as if their flashlight batteries are being run down. Their light gets dimmer, and they don't know what's wrong. If we deny them the time, space, and

Hours spent alone in quiet provide a necessary lull in the rhythm of the day.

flexibility they need to develop at their own pace, they will not be able to recharge their batteries.

The ancient Chinese philosopher Lao Tzu reminds us that "it is not the clay the potter throws that gives the jar its usefulness, but the space within." If stimulation and guidance are the clay, then time by oneself is the space within. Hours spent alone in daydreams or in quiet, unstructured activities – preferably out in nature – instill a sense of security and independence and provide a necessary lull in the rhythm of the day. Children thrive on silence. Without external distractions, they will often become so inspired by what they are doing that they will be totally oblivious of everything around them. Unfortunately, silence is such a luxury that they are rarely allowed the opportunity for such undisturbed concentration.

As parents and caregivers, how can we find creative ways to give children more silence and space? In schools, some teachers stand at the classroom door with a bag, confiscating all phones and tablets for the duration of the class so that children can focus. Others send home letters to parents requesting less entertainment time after school hours. They point out that children are more likely to get their homework done and have a good night's sleep.

Image from Kay Polk

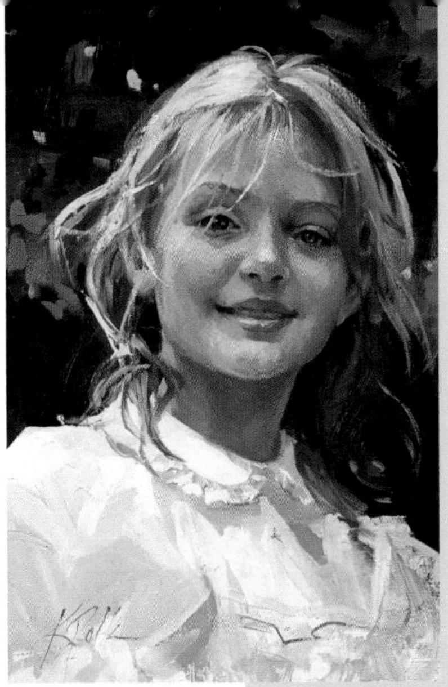

In Los Altos, California, children of Google, Apple, and Hewlett-Packard executives attend a Waldorf School that doesn't use computers in the classroom. If executives in the world of high technology choose a school that protects their children from computers, other parents and teachers need to hear about it. But even if schools are unwilling to scrap their much-bragged-about technology, there are outdoor programs that can do wonders for a child's confidence. Sometimes, all children need is a chance to find out for themselves that the real world is more interesting than the virtual world.

White space and nature can be healing for troubled children. But, like most remedies, they work better if taken preventatively. We can proactively make changes before things get desperate. Can you do without a television? Thousands of families do, with heartening results. Having grown up without one, I found it easier to leave it out of my own home, sparing our children the advertising that would relentlessly inform them, among other things, of further advanced technology that they "just had to have."

If several nearby families opt for freedom from screens, it can become a groundswell movement. Children can play together and adults won't feel as if they're the only ones out of step with the times.

In my house, as in many, computers are merely tools for adults to do their work; we don't turn to them for entertainment. My kids only learned typing in middle school, when

Insight

FRIEDRICH FROEBEL

WE GRANT SPACE and time to young plants and animals because we know that, in accordance with the laws that live in them, they will develop properly and grow well. Young animals and plants are given rest, and arbitrary interference with their growth is avoided, because it is known that the opposite practice would disturb their pure unfolding and sound development. But the young human being is looked upon as a piece of wax, a lump of clay which we can mold into whatever we please. You, who roam through garden and field, through meadow and grove, why do you close your mind to the silent teaching of nature? Behold even the weed, which, grown up amid hindrances and constraint, scarcely yields an indication of inner law; behold it in nature, in field or garden, and see how perfectly it conforms to law – what a pure inner life it shows, harmonious in all parts and features; a beautiful sun, a radiant star, it has burst from the earth! Thus, O parents, could your children, on whom you force in tender years forms and aims against their nature, and who, therefore, walk with you in morbid and unnatural deformity – thus could your children, too, unfold in beauty and develop in all-sided harmony!

Friedrich Froebel, who created the concept of the kindergarten, was a reformist nineteenth-century educator who emphasized the value of teaching the "whole child" through active play, creativity, music, art, and hands-on learning. froebelweb.org

Source: *The Education of Man* (New York: D. Appleton and Co., 1906), 8–9.

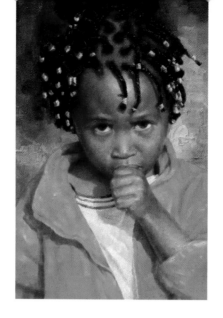

their term papers were long enough to warrant the effort. Parents can support their children's research, teaming up for internet searches if they're required, but also taking library trips together and swapping books. It's a great chance to point out that anyone can say anything online, but that doesn't mean it's true.

World news should be a part of a child's education, but it does not need to be accompanied by graphic images. It is hard enough for us adults to process the pain and suffering we see in the news each day without becoming jaded or allowing it to harden our hearts. If adults take the time to read up on current events or listen to public radio, we can approach difficult subjects in a way that respects a child's age and understanding. This can provide an opening for further discussion about world suffering and what can be done to alleviate it.

The catch, of course, is our own time. In our over-scheduled adult lives, we're not sure we have time to work and play together with our kids, or sit and talk about the news. But when

> *Let's tune in to the living, breathing wonders who are waiting for us to look up and notice them.*

we think of the alternatives, it is worth making time, and making it now. We only have these few years together. Society may lament an epidemic of lost, cynical teens, incapable of compassion or empathy. But if children's spirits aren't guided and protected by those closest to them, what do we expect?

It's time for us to take a hard look at all the clever devices in our own lives that everyone calls timesavers. When we sit texting on a playground bench while our kids play alone, whose time are we saving? When we send one more tweet, read one more article, play one more round of a video game while children are in the vicinity, we're telling them that something else is more important than they are. We can talk about children's technological addictions all we want, but the problem starts closer to home.

Let's put our machines away and tune in to the living, breathing wonders who are waiting for us to notice them. Let's shut off the power, take our child by the hand, and show him that the real world is a fascinating place. ⤳

This article was excerpted from Johann Christoph Arnold's book Their Name Is Today *(Plough, 2014).* plough.com/theirnameistoday

Photograph by De Visu / Big Stock

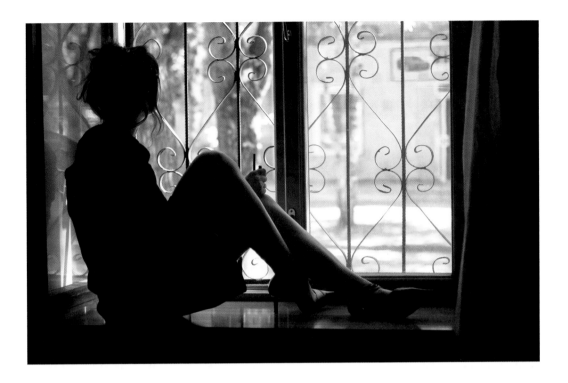

The Technology of Gender
Examining an Unsettled Science

AN INTERVIEW WITH PAUL R. McHUGH

Future technologies, we're told, will allow humankind to literally reshape who we are – for instance, by editing our own DNA or connecting our brains directly to computer networks. While such possibilities give ample cause for alarm, in fact we're already using technology to modify human bodies: through sex reassignment. This package of hormonal treatment and radical plastic surgeries is finding ever-increasing social acceptance. But what's at

Dr. Paul R. McHugh is professor of psychiatry at Johns Hopkins University, where from 1975 to 2001 he was department chair as well as psychiatrist-in-chief at Johns Hopkins Hospital. Dr. McHugh is author of several books including The Mind Has Mountains: Reflections on Society and Psychiatry *(Johns Hopkins, 2008).*

stake when we artificially alter a human being in regard to something as fundamental as biological sex? *Plough* spoke to Paul McHugh, professor of psychiatry at the Johns Hopkins School of Medicine, about his experience treating children and adolescents with gender dysphoria.

Plough: *What has your research revealed about hormone treatments for children?*

Dr. McHugh: We reviewed all the proposals and mechanisms about how these hormones might work in children with gender dysphoria, and there's no evidence that this treatment leads to happy results. Experimental treatments like this ordinarily go with a set of standard accompaniments. First, they go through an Institutional Review Board (IRB). It became clear in the 1940s and 1950s that many hospitals were using patients as experimental subjects without their consent. To avoid that, IRBs were established. Patients need to give fully informed consent: the doctor needs to say, "we're doing an experiment on you; we hope the results will be good, but we don't know."

Second, the treatment groups need to be checked against comparison groups. And finally, there needs to be detailed, long-term follow-up. But these hormone treatments are now considered standard of care without any of this being done. There is no good evidence that this is a beneficial treatment. There are testimonials, but that's not the same. And at the moment there are no proper studies on it.

What can you tell us about the children who are seeking these treatments?

Many of these children have been drawn into this idea, that they are "really" the opposite sex, through the internet. They've got very vigorous social media support. They run on testimonials and trust. The young people are very vulnerable to that; they go on the internet and hear things they trust. They go to their parents and say, "I want to do this," but this is the same age that you wouldn't dream of letting anybody have a

tattoo. It's a craze-like phenomenon, and now it's on the increase, especially among young women. It's very much like anorexia nervosa or body dysmorphic disorder; they're absolutely committed to living in this way and they resent anyone who doesn't support them in it.

I'm beset with families calling me: "Where can we get someone to help us, given that we're being asked to collaborate in making this permanent change happen?" They're very distressed.

In 2016 you coauthored a 145-page study on gender and sexuality (see "Further Reading" opposite). How was the report received? It was controversial in the popular press . . .

On a scientific level, there was no explosive challenge. It almost sank without notice. You would think that people would respond with counterclaims, contrary research: that there is good evidence for these hormone treatments being beneficial. But that didn't happen. Nobody said solid experimental evidence existed.

What are doctors' responsibilities here?

Proposing a future different from what nature would recommend is a huge problem. Here's something that's so obviously against nature, and it fits into other things that are against nature, like assisted suicide. Doctors used to be in the position of helping nature, helping the body heal, but now it's different. Political pressures are so great. We're called transphobic: how could we be phobic toward these kids? The presumption is that we're acting in bad faith for them. But we, and their parents, want to help them and benefit them; we don't want to be responsible in the long run for injuries done to them.

What do you expect will happen with this in the future?

This is early times for us now. We expect that the regrets will start coming, but we're not sure how to help. The best thing to do for these young people is to postpone any physical change, any physical intervention. Maybe the best course of action is to ask someone to live as the opposite sex without doing anything physical. But this is very difficult, and the children are so convinced that they want a sex change that they threaten to do themselves injury. It's an unprecedented kind of treatment to be done on young people, because there's no evidence that it has good long-term effects.

What do you know about long-term prospects of resolution for gender dysphoria if these hormone treatments aren't administered?

Again, we know very little. University of Toronto researcher Dr. Kenneth Zucker worked with twenty-five girls who were experiencing feelings of gender incongruence, using family therapy among other things, and – crucially – treating co-occurring psychological disorders that were contributing to these girls' distress. He treated gender dysphoria as an idiom of distress, rather than an entity in itself, and sought to address any co-occurring psychological issues.

In a follow-up study after thirty years, twenty-three of the twenty-five girls had resolved their feelings of gender incongruence. Other studies indicate that these feelings resolve in 80 percent of cases as the young people grow up. But we just don't really know, we don't have good studies, and crucially, we are not doing comparative treatments. All we'll have, in the next couple of years, is the outcome of this phenomenal experiment. And I expect that regret will run high. ➤

FOR FURTHER READING

"Sexuality and Gender: Findings from the Biological, Psychological, and Social Sciences"
Lawrence S. Mayer and Paul R. McHugh
New Atlantis, Fall 2016, no. 50

What is sexual orientation? How do we understand transgenderism? And what is the role of medicine and biotechnology in addressing these issues? The answers to questions like these touch on some of the most personally and politically fraught issues of the day. In 2016, the *New Atlantis,* a journal of technology and society, published a lengthy report by Drs. Lawrence S. Mayer and Paul R. McHugh, both of Johns Hopkins University. This report approaches questions related to gender and sexuality by surveying available research across several disciplines. The authors' conclusion? It's complicated. The report challenges some of the dominant ideas surrounding these issues: sexual orientation is neither a choice nor a fixed and inborn trait, they say, with causes that are incompletely understood.

When it comes to transgenderism, the authors speak more strongly: the claim that a human being can change his or her sex "is starkly, nakedly false," says Dr. McHugh. The practice of blocking puberty or administering hormones to children who identify as a member of the opposite sex, say Mayer and McHugh, has no therapeutic merit. The report concludes that "more effort is called for to provide people [who are personally wrestling with these issues] with the understanding, care, and support they need to lead healthy, flourishing lives." ➤

The Editors

Download the complete report at *thenewatlantis.com.*

Digging Deeper

HOW TO THINK WELL ABOUT TECHNOLOGY

Writers have long wrestled with the question of how the machines we shape in turn shape us. Since at least the nineteenth century, with its intense awareness of (and anxiety about) technological change, novels and works of nonfiction have attempted to grapple with the questions of how the technology we use influences us and how we can best understand and respond to its advances. Some of the most enduring of these books are below.

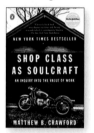 **Matthew Crawford's** 2010 book, *Shop Class as Soulcraft: An Inquiry into the Value of Work* (Penguin Books) is in many ways a love letter to good technology. Crawford shows how working on motorcycles draws him out of his head – in fact, a follow-up book, also well worth your while, is called *The World Beyond Your Head: On Becoming an Individual in an Age of Distraction* – and embeds him in the physical world. He leads readers, even those who aren't motorcycle aficionados, to see the tasks of engineering and repairing as deeply human endeavors, ones that break down the apparent gap between thinking and doing. To be able to repair is to have a kind of power, and a motorcycle mechanic has a very concrete role in a community, one that can't be outsourced. Crawford's arguments aren't abstract: he makes them as he tells his own story. The book is a memoir as well as a reflection, and the author's love for both the work he does and the people who've enabled him to do it are apparent on every page.

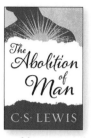 **C. S. Lewis's** *The Abolition of Man* (HarperOne) is a short, sane, and shocking book. It's about how children should be educated and how education differs from conditioning. It's about morality and how to understand the idea that a moral world exists outside of human convenience and utility. But it's also about technology. Absent an understanding of the Good, says Lewis, our power over nature through technology ultimately destroys everything that makes us distinctly human. We gain greater power with technological and biotechnological tools, but we believe ourselves, and nature, to be reduced to what those tools can manipulate. Finally, human beings cease to understand themselves as people: "They are not men at all: they are artifacts. Man's final conquest has proved to be the abolition of man."

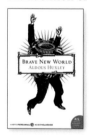 **Aldous Huxley's** classic dystopian novel *Brave New World* (Harper Perennial) is, in certain ways, the fictional working out of Lewis's worst-case scenario. In the society it portrays, domination of the natural world and of the human self is near-complete. A futuristic society in which a commitment to the mass-production techniques of Henry Ford has replaced Christianity provides the backdrop for the struggles of those who haven't entirely succumbed to the reshaping of the world. Bioengineering has separated society into castes, but there is no real social unrest, because all castes have access

to drugs that simulate happiness. There is no romance or marriage, but there's plenty of sex. With no challenges to overcome, there's no possibility of failure. "A really efficient totalitarian state," writes Huxley, "would be one in which a population of slaves . . . do not have to be coerced, because they love their servitude." Against that servitude, Huxley's novel stands as a call for vigilance.

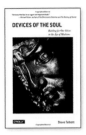

Steve Talbott's *Devices of the Soul: Battling for Our Selves in the Age of Machines* (O'Reilly Media) deserves to be better known. A series of essays covering many aspects of the human encounter with technology, this work is not technophobic – but it is profoundly cautious. Talbott brings a uniquely thoughtful approach to topics that range from the allure of modern hunting weapons for Amazon tribesmen to the impoverishment of education that results when computers are adopted as primary teaching tools, and from the perils of efficiency to Silicon Valley's breathless paeans to the possibility of artificial consciousness. The influence of his interest in the work of Rudolf Steiner is apparent, but his reflections are interestingly congruent with those a Christian might make. Talbott urges us, above all, to be more thoughtful about our adoption of technology. "I don't think modern technology necessarily alienates us from the world it mediates," he says. "But a lot depends on our recognizing how it can do so."

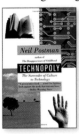

Neil Postman's *Technopoly: The Surrender of Culture to Technology* (Vintage) is a new classic of techno-criticism, and the author's trademark wit makes the book a pleasure to read. Technology, he emphasizes, is not a neutral tool to be used to further the goals of an existing culture; rather, it shapes a culture's goals. The mechanical clock, for example, invented to keep track of the hours of prayer in Benedictine monasteries, shaped the way we perceive time and eventually allowed the birth of the highly organized factory system of production: "In the eternal struggle between God and Mammon, the clock quite unpredictably favored the latter." The scientific revolution and especially the nineteenth century saw the birth of a culture of technocracy. More and more, the purpose of the world was to be found in applying increasingly elaborate technologies to the utilitarian solution of human problems. Contemporary America, Postman claims, is the world's first technopoly – a totalitarian technocracy. His solution? Be a "loving resistance fighter." Retain the humane and (though he is not a conventional believer) religious values that help us decide not just how to do something but what it is that we should do. ✎ *The Editors*

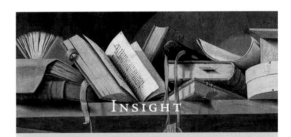

INSIGHT

The machine yes the machine
Never wastes anybody's time
Never watches the foreman
Never talks back
Never says what is right or wrong
The machine yes the machine
Cuts your production costs
A man is a man and what can you do with him?
A man is a man and what can you do with him?

Carl Sandburg

The Gods *of* Progress

PHILIP BRITTS

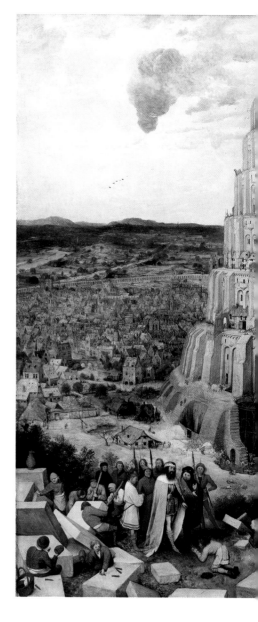

NEVER MORE SO than now, the myth of progress remains the story by which we live our lives. Every disruption and new product rollout reinforces it. But where are we progressing to? In 1948, just as the postwar technological boom began, the English farmer-poet Philip Britts penned this essay on what he called "spiritual evolution."

ARE WE STANDING at the beginning of a new age of scientific development, of supersonic speeds, of atomic energy, of more and more wonderful machines? Or are we standing, unaware, at the end of the machine age, at the end of the progress of scientific power? Are we about to enter an era of greater wealth, greater luxury, greater leisure, the modern home, people emancipated from drudgery? Or has this age of power reached its climax, and will this civilization destroy itself with those forces that it has created?

To reject this question, to sail onward in the arrogant confidence that man can and will manipulate these tremendous forces for the good of all, is to put more pressure on the drift to catastrophe. Is not this the poison of the age, the belief of man in man? "Man is certainly stark mad," said Montaigne, "He cannot make a

Philip Britts (1917–1949) was a horticulturalist and poet (see biographical note on page 46).

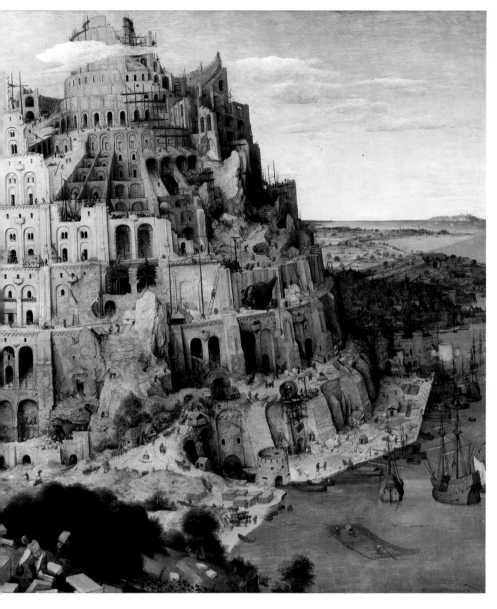

Pieter Bruegel
the Elder,
*Construction
of the
Tower of Babel,*
1563

flea, and yet he will be making gods by dozens."

Yet many people have the question in their hearts, and many, many people are haunted by the fear of another war. . . . All this leads to a further question: Is man himself making spiritual progress; is he, together with his indisputable intellectual enlightenment, becoming a more noble creature?

Today man can speak and his voice be carried instantaneously to a hundred million listeners, thousands of miles apart – but has

he anything to say that is more vital for the welfare of humanity than what Isaiah, or Plato, proclaimed with the unaided voice?

Let it never be denied that sometimes a word of shining wisdom is spoken and printed. There is gold amongst the dross. But if one speaks of mankind making progress, one speaks and dreams of mankind as a whole: in one's mind is a vision of the human race, very gradually, and perhaps even with up-and-down spirals, but very gradually, as a race, rising to nobler heights.

Against this conception of man's spiritual evolution a mountain of evidence is piling up, more than could be put into many volumes of heavy books. Some things have been greatly publicized: the concentration camps, lynchings in the US, the rapidly increasing divorce rates, the bombing of Hiroshima, and the continued manufacture of atomic bombs in the postwar armaments race.

> **There is a skeleton in our cupboard – the skeleton of an ape.**

But those who put their trust in progress reply that these horrors that mar our civilization are committed by a relative few. The average man is more enlightened, kindlier, more humane than his remoter forbears. Progress is slow, and sometimes interrupted by the backsliding of a certain race. On the whole, though, we have made great strides in education, and in the care of the mentally and physically diseased, and in our provisions for social relief. We have definitely become more social-conscious. We have . . . done great things in organization and collaboration.

And there are these veins of gold in the mental output of the world. It would be hard to say if they are more than formerly, or are increasing, but they are more efficiently disseminated. They reach a better educated public, they come from better educated minds. Still it doesn't seem to be invariably so that the sublimest truths are uttered by the best-trained minds, and it would be hard to prove that the gold is purer than it was in the past.

"Be ye all like-minded, compassionate, loving as brethren, tender-hearted, humble-minded." This was written by a fisherman in the year 63. Has anything more valuable to mankind been said by any philosopher or theologian in the twentieth century?

Strangely enough, it isn't so much by looking at other people around us that we have become so convinced of this upward trend of humanity. Conviction is carried most strongly home to our heart by looking at ourselves. . . . We feel deep within us that, however imperfect we are, we are humane and kindly people. We are seekers for truth, and we live according to our lights. We have our ideals, and we strive to be an influence for good in the world.

There is a skeleton in our cupboard – the skeleton of an ape. Half of our restless pressing onward, half of our so frantically clothing ourselves with knowledge, culture, civilization, is caused by our need to fly from the skeleton of this ancestral ape. . . . And in the course of our progress we commit atrocities more hideous than any of nature's cruelest beasts could dream of. The character of the beast of prey dominates world society, a beast of prey not only empowered with tremendous physical

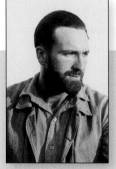

Philip Britts (1917–1949) was a farmer, poet, and mystic. Born in Devon, England, his search for a way of life where people could work together in harmony with nature and one another led him to join the Bruderhof just before the beginning of the Second World War. As pacifists, he and his wife Joan left England in 1941 for the Bruderhof in Paraguay. While working as a horticulturalist, he contracted the tropical disease that would take his life at the age of thirty-one, leaving Joan with three young children and a fourth on the way.

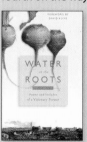

Philip's essays and poetry are featured in an upcoming book, *Water at the Roots: Poems and Insights of a Visionary Farmer,* ed. Jennifer Harries (Plough, March 2018). The article above is excerpted from this book.

resources, but empowered with a highly trained intellect to serve his malicious ends.

Or perhaps the beast is alive within us. There is no possibility of leaving him behind, of climbing to peaks he cannot reach. There is the alternative of fight or submit to his rule. But within us also, or rather, ready to enter every open heart, is the spirit that fights against the beast, the spirit of the New Man. And the fight is a choice, with which we are faced every day, and in which we have free will to choose: Which spirit shall I serve?

Our only choice is a choice of service. All our sparkling ability, our insight, our psycho-physical resources, are drawn into the service of one or the other. . . . We are free to choose. But let us beware of trying to choose both.

In absolute opposition to what we have been calling the spirit of the beast is the spirit of love. This spirit alone can bring that peace which is in absolute opposition to war and death and destruction. Peace that is born of love and filled with love is the only true peace. It is not just a cessation of war, a shaking of the ripe fruit while the tree goes on growing to bear again in due season. Peace can only arise when the tree is cut down and rooted out. In this mighty work, love uses weapons that are in absolute opposition to the weapons of the beast. Instead of the good man, the poor in spirit; instead of the confidence in the progress of man, the sorrowful recognition of the helplessness of man; instead of the mighty, the meek; instead of self-satisfaction, the hunger-ing and thirsting for righteousness; instead of judgement, mercy; instead of the doctrine of many paths, singleness and pureness of heart; instead of coercion, reconciliation; instead of success, persecution for righteousness' sake.

Against the multiple weapons of division, love constructs the fortress of unity. This, too,

has its foundations way down in the practical things of daily life. Mine and thine are done away with, in material as in spiritual things. Property divides men, the haves from the have-nots-or-not-so-much. It is one of the first barriers that melts in the glow of love. But individual pride and self-respect are properties of the heart. They vanish too, in the realization that we are all weak men, and there is none good but God; that we are all brothers and one is our master, even Christ. We are no longer separated individuals, each with a slightly different "kingdom of God" within us. But we are all members of one body, with a common purpose and a common source of strength to follow it. Thus each shares with the other, goods and work and table, for everything belongs to the spirit of love. Each helps the other, and accepts help, for the victory is not unto us. There arises brotherhood, as the true calling of man, as the fruit of the spirit of love, as the unity that establishes peace.

There is always this insistence of Jesus upon deeds, not words. Even the cup of water to the least of these my brethren. One drop of lifeblood spent in the actual practice of brotherhood is more effec-tive in the struggle for peace than an ocean of ink written about it. This would not be true perhaps if victory lay within the power of man, if the struggle were one of human goodwill against human weakness, of human progress against our obscure origins; if the kingdom of God could be set up by man. The faith that an ounce of action is worth a ton of speech, the faith that there can be any significance what-ever in a tiny group of very ordinary people trying to live in brotherhood, can rest only on the faith in the living God. That God acts, and that his will is love, his purpose peace on the earth, is the justification for the decision to put

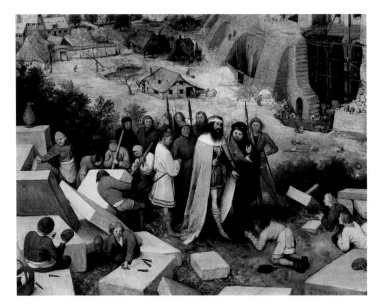

that will wholly into practice in our lives here and now. It is the significance of the savor of the salt. The vital thing is not the bulk of the substance, but that the salt be salt.

Community is not a system solving the economic-social question.

Community is not a system for solving the economic-social problem. Many such communities have been organized and have failed to stay the course. Community is a consequence. Community is the consequence of people being kindled with the glow of love. Community is the consequence when people see right through to the depths the necessity of the fundamental choice: either-or. Either unity or division, either brotherhood or war. It is when people see this choice and, having seen it, make the choice to serve the spirit of love in terms of unconditional surrender, that they are drawn together, that they are given community through the power of love. A new form of society emerges because men are filled with a new spirit. Community cannot exist in the absence of the spirit of love. Love cannot be expressed where there is division, competition, isolation, egotism. Each one must give himself wholeheartedly to all – making no reservations.

"The kingdom of God is within you." This sentence has been twisted by the religion of this world to blind us to the real and concrete issues. The kingdom of God is not a comfortable feeling inside that we have attained a harmony of our souls with abstract truth. Above all, the kingdom of God is not the private property of each individual soul. The kingdom of God is the reign of God on this earth. To the words, "Thy kingdom come," belong the words, "Thy will be done on earth. . . ." The powers of the kingdom of God are at work wherever division is overcome by unity, wherever barriers are swept away by brotherhood.

Instead of the glittering palace of manifold divisions, let us seek a simple house with an open door. Instead of the towering organization of worldly skill and worldly knowledge, let us seek a humble trust in God. Let us make the unconditional surrender to the spirit of love. "Except a man be born again he cannot enter the kingdom of heaven." Let us beware of trying to save ourselves by going the two ways. "He who seeks his life shall lose it." Are we standing at the brink of long vistas of prosperous evolution, or is civilization moving towards its own destruction? Has it the seeds of life or death within it? Our only choice is a choice of service, and service means deed, not word. It is either-or. Serve one or the other. Prune the great tree of division or plant the new tree of brotherhood. Let us not be misled by the symptoms of human power. The power of God alone is decisive in the end. ➤

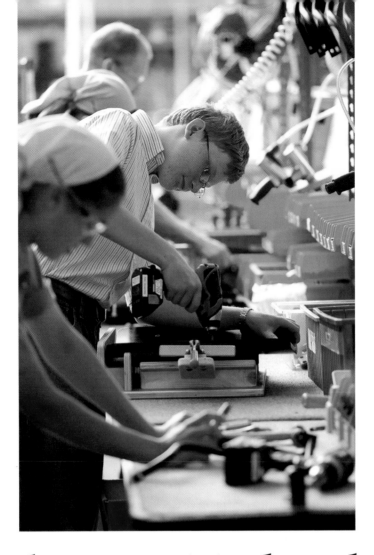

Anabaptist Technology

Lessons from a Communitarian Business

JOHN RHODES

In 1998, Community Playthings, the church-run manufacturing business based in New York in which I work, tried abandoning email. This was not my idea, despite the fact that I'd been leading the company for five years. Instead, the impetus for the move came from the company's staff. Many of them were angry about the effects email was having.

Today it may seem quaint that people once regarded email, that clunky relic of a time before social media, as a threatening technology. Yet the workers' complaints were real enough. Email, they felt, exacerbated tensions between colleagues, who used it to bypass each other when making decisions or to avoid resolving conflicts face to face. In what had

Young and old, skilled and unskilled, work together in a community workshop.

John Rhodes is director of development for Community Playthings and Rifton Equipment.

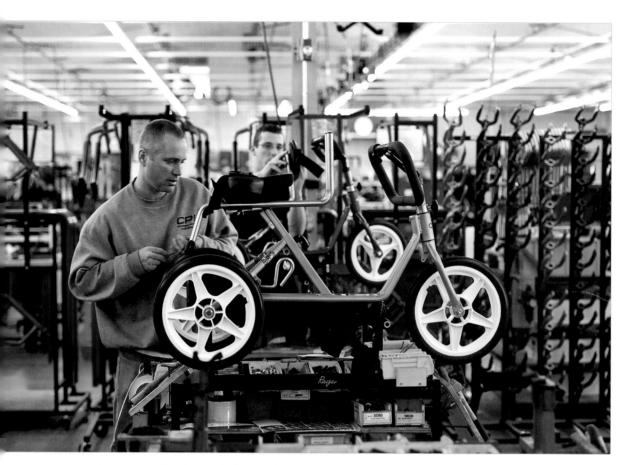

Working together in harmony is fundamental to Bruderhof businesses.

been an egalitarian workplace with a strong emphasis on collaboration, it erected a divide between those who enjoyed constant access to instant communication because they worked at a computer, and those without such access because they were busy building the wooden toys and furniture we sold. The management team, too, noticed how email led to time waste as office workers were distracted from their duties by recreational listservs devoted to news or sports. (Yes, this was once a thing.) All in all, with the advent of email something had changed in our company. Even I, a supporter of technological business applications who had worked on developing computerized systems since the 1970s, had to admit that it wasn't all for the better.

Community Playthings' particular culture made this situation especially painful. Founded in 1948 by communitarian pacifists in Georgia, since the 1950s the company has been the main source of income and work for the members of the Bruderhof, a Christian community movement in the Anabaptist tradition whose members share all things in common in the spirit of the early church (Acts 2 and 4). All those who work in the company are my fellow Bruderhof members; in keeping with our vow of personal poverty, none of us owns a share or earns a paycheck, with all earnings going to support the community or to fund its philanthropic and missionary projects.

Despite its communal context, Community Playthings has thrived in the capitalist marketplace. Along with Rifton Equipment, another community-run company that makes therapeutic equipment for people with disabilities, it sells to customers around the world; in 1998, earnings were covering all costs for two thousand people in eight Bruderhof locations in the United States and Europe. Both companies, though medium-sized in terms of market share, are recognized as industry leaders for their durable products and vanguard designs. Such success sprang at least in part from our adoption of innovative technologies. The company had computerized already in 1979, buying a Wang minicomputer; a decade later, a second growth spurt resulted from adopting the Japanese "Just-in-Time" manufacturing philosophy, which made extensive use of manufacturing data.

The fundamental secret of Community Playthings, however, is our commitment to working together with everyone else in the business in a spirit of harmony. Deeply ingrained in our company culture is an abhorrence of any corporate hierarchy. Since the purpose of the company is simply to be an extension of our common life in Christian community, we are brothers and sisters, not managers and employees. While some individuals obviously carry leadership responsibility, all of us earn the same pay: nothing. In the words of Bruderhof founder Eberhard Arnold, "love is joy in others," and this love is to pervade all we do, even at the cost of business efficiency. True to this ethos, the company needs to accommodate a wide range of workers: young and old, female and male, able-bodied and less so, skilled and unskilled, lifelong community member and newcomer.

Up until the late 1990s, bringing new technologies into the business had rarely been controversial. The office staff, especially, applauded anything that reduced the drudgery of repetitive typing. Previously, the main worries had focused on the introduction of CNC (computer numeric control) machines to production – some older members had raised questions about the loss of old-school craftsmanship and the sudden importance of the machines' young tech-savvy operators.

But it was email that proved to be the bridge too far. Frustration with the unintended consequences of electronic communication mounted, and before long there were proposals for an enterprise-wide email ban. For those of us charged with steering a complex multi-locational operation, with a number of business processes dependent on the email system, we definitely had a "Houston, we have a problem" moment.

Technology is never neutral: once introduced, it plays its hand.

In conversations with my fellow members, I acknowledged that email was a technology with low emotional bandwidth: excellent for sharing information, poor or even often awful at creating and sustaining warmth in relationships. But I argued that in a communication-rich environment, where we lived and worked together, met face to face daily for communal meals and worship, and shared a commitment to avoid all gossip and backbiting, email's weaknesses should be manageable.

The fact that this isn't how it played out taught me a valuable lesson: technology is never neutral. As the French thinker Jacques Ellul recognized, the technologies we use always have an effect on us, and that effect is both burden and blessing. Importantly, the outcome of a given form of technology depends less on our intent than on the structure of that technology. Once introduced, it plays its hand. Our task is to keep our eyes open and understand what is happening.

This is no easy task, for the changes wrought by technology are often subtle and unpredictable. They can affect our very concept of life and our place in it. Neil Postman, in his book

Technopoly, gives an example of how this happens:

> Who would have imagined, for example, whose interests and what worldview would be ultimately advanced by the invention of the mechanical clock? The clock had its origin in the Benedictine monasteries of the twelfth and thirteenth centuries. The impetus behind the invention was to provide a more or less precise regularity to the routines of the monasteries, which required, among other things, seven periods of devotion during the course of the day. The bells of the monastery were to be rung to signal the canonical hours; the mechanical clock was the technology that could provide precision to these rituals of devotion. And indeed, it did. But what the monks did not foresee was that the clock is a means not merely of keeping track of the hours but also of synchronizing and controlling the actions of men. And thus, by the middle of the fourteenth century, the clock had moved outside the walls of the monastery, and brought a new and precise regularity to the life of the workman and the merchant.
>
> "The mechanical clock," as Lewis Mumford wrote, "made possible the idea of regular production, regular working hours and a standardized product." In short, without the clock, capitalism would have been quite impossible. The paradox, the surprise, and the wonder are that the clock was invented by men who wanted to devote themselves more rigorously to God; it ended as the technology of greatest use to men who wished to devote themselves to the accumulation of money.[1]

Unintended consequences are not the only effect of technology. As Postman argues, it is not possible to contain the effects of technology to a limited sphere of human activity – "one significant change generates total change."

The solution is not a legalistic retreat into traditionalism.

He gives a string of examples to illustrate the point: "If you remove the caterpillars from a given habitat, you are not left with the same environment minus caterpillars. You have a new environment, and have reconstituted the conditions of survival. The same is true if you add caterpillars to an environment that has none." Likewise, in 1500, "fifty years after the printing press was invented, we did not have old Europe plus the printing press. We had a different Europe." The same was true after the invention of the automobile, radio, television, and every other major technology. This inevitable effect, and the uncertainty of this effect, is what makes us so uneasy about new technology.

As our company debated how to use electronic communication, I found myself making heavy use of Postman's book, which distills the thought of dozens of earlier thinkers on technology including Ellul, Ivan Illich, and Marshall McLuhan. Given our company's context as part of a Christian community, I found Postman's account of the spiritual history of technology especially illuminating. Prior to the seventeenth century, he argues, most cultures found a way to integrate technology into an existing pattern of life rather than be taken over by it. Often, those cultures that possessed the strongest philosophical or religious center were also best able to pull off this feat of integration: where people were confident that their existence had meaning and order, it was "almost impossible for technics to subordinate [them] to its own needs." Technological developments brought about changes, some significant, but still the culture's values and institutions guided inventions and limited their effects.

Francis Bacon, however, heralded a new attitude when he wrote in his 1620 masterwork

Photograph by Mark McCarty, courtesy of Rifton

Novum Organum that the only goal of science is the "endowment of human life with new inventions and riches." Progress, with its emphasis on efficiency and production, was born. By the end of the next century, the factory system was developed, Postman writes, and "small-scale, personalized, skilled labor" gave way to "large-scale, impersonal, mechanized production." Our concept of human nature began to shift. People were no longer children of God, but economic units, treated like machines during work, and as consumers otherwise.

It was technology's tendency toward dehumanization, I realized, that my fellow community members were reacting to in their objections to email. While profoundly inconvenient for those of us leading the business, the reaction was a healthy one, rooted in our community's tradition. Eberhard Arnold, in laying the groundwork for the Bruderhof's structure in the 1920s and 1930s, addressed the subject of technology extensively. Having seen firsthand the dehumanization of factory workers, he was skeptical of its benefits: "Many machines do not permit man to put his soul, his heart, his mind into the work; it is a curse for man to have to do something without having his whole heart in it."[2] He was horrified that Christians passively accepted technology's evils, such as the tens of thousands of traffic deaths that accompanied the spread of automobiles.

Yet to Arnold, the solution was not a legalistic retreat into traditionalism. Instead, he insisted on recovering the old integration of technology into a holistic vision for how humans can best flourish. As he wrote in 1921:

> We cannot yet tell in detail how this communal love of work with its voluntary nature and joy in creativity will become practical reality. We do not know to what extent mechanized industry will be struck when the works of the

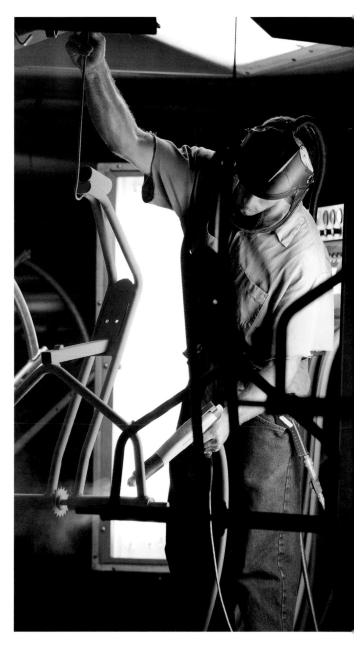

> devil are destroyed. The evolution of work has arrived at a deadlock: division of labor and victimization of people. Love must also become inventive in the technical area, so that soul, oversight, and unity are brought into every piece of work once more.[3]

Technology is integrated into community life, but does not dominate it.

Technology has found its rightful place, then, when it enables people to work well with all faculties of their being, and to work well with one another.

ommunity Playthings' email crisis soon passed. After a week or two of email sabbath, we cautiously began using it again, now with a common awareness of dangers to avoid and a renewed commitment not to allow barriers to grow between us. Two decades later, email is regarded as outdated. Yet the principles we learned from this episode have continued to guide our communities in the years since, and not just in business life. Here are four of them:

1. *Families and community first.* Any use of technology that undermines the richness of human relationships is presumed suspect, especially technologies that encourage passivity rather than creativity. That's why Bruderhof members minimize their use of social media, and why Bruderhof homes don't have television. It's not that we regard either of these as a sin; it's just that we've seen how it distracts from more important ways to spend our time, such as reading a book to a child, inviting a lonely neighbor over for tea, or painting a picture. For similar reasons, we seek to push back against the pressure, enabled by technology, to allow our daytime work to spill over into times that should be reserved for our families or for the community. The laptops stay in the office when five o'clock rolls around.

2. *Technologies have an agenda.* Often the agenda is that of mammon: many technologies are designed to turn us into consumers. (Television, again, is a timeworn but still relevant example.) Since this is the case, we ought to approach them with the same skepticism we'd show an untrustworthy used-car salesman. As Postman points out, it's the structure of the technology, not our intentions in using it, which often change us most.

3. *Screens and children don't mix.* This is a corollary of points 1 and 2. For several years,

Bruderhof schools enthusiastically adopted educational technology. The results were alarming, and our communities did an about-turn, removing computers from the classroom up to high school. The reason: the heart of education is not the transfer of knowledge, but the nurturing of relationships – of child to teacher, of children among each other, and of children to nature. Academic learning, while important, takes second place to the more central educational task of growing in relationships, and in fact often occurs as a side benefit to it. In this process, the intrusion of a machine is counterproductive. (Quite different is the use of technologies for children with disabilities, for example communication boards for those who cannot speak. Rather than substituting for relationships, such technologies make them possible.)

4. *Don't be afraid to walk away.* To be tech-savvy is not a virtue; "blessed are the early adopters" is not a wise rule for living. If a form of technology is proving to be deleterious to relationships with others, we must have the fortitude to drop it.

At times, as in our community's abortive attempt to get rid of email, we'll end up reversing course, either adopting a new technology that we've spurned or re-adopting one we tried to do without. Even then, the exercise of sorting out the good effects from the bad is almost always a fruitful one. It ensures that we are technology's master, with our tools serving to promote human flourishing – not the other way around. ⤙

1. Neil Postman, *Technopoly: The Surrender of Culture to Technology* (Vintage, 1993), 15. The following three paragraphs draw extensively on Postman's book.

2. Eberhard Arnold, "The Problem of Machines," talk given on August 8, 1935, trans. Nicoline Maas and Hela Ehrlich (Bruderhof Historical Archive, EA 439).

3. Eberhard Arnold, "Community and the Future of Work," unpublished manuscript, 1921, trans. Emmy Barth Maendel (Bruderhof Historical Archive, EA 20/21a).

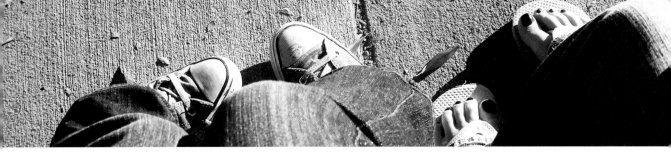

Your Neighbor Lives Next Door

The Computer-Free Way to Happiness

CHICO FAJARDO-HEFLIN

When my wife and I unpacked our boxes in our new home in the crumbling town of Ford Heights, Illinois, nine years ago, one thing we did not have to unpack was a computer. Unnerved by how wired our lives were becoming, Tatiana and I had begun untangling ourselves from technology we thought we'd be better off without. The microwave was the first to go. Then went the dishwasher, followed by the lawnmower, car, and cell phone. We swore off transportation by air, and then, finally, we pulled the plug on the computer.

When folks ask us what it's like to live without many of the conveniences of modern technology, our best answer is that it has localized our lives. Without email and Facebook, we must nurture most of our relationships in person. This has meant that, while we have lost contact with hundreds of former friends, we know nearly every person on our block. Without access to blogs and news websites, we are out of touch with the latest presidential tweet, but we do know when a neighbor runs out of medication. Without air travel, conferences and edgy gatherings of "radicals" are mostly out of the question, but we can attest to the great joy that a neighborhood bonfire brings. Though scaling down our world from across the country to across the street has been challenging, it has helped us root ourselves more deeply in this place.

Some of you are protesting that you, too, are aware when your neighbor's medication runs out. Even now, you are ordering a refill for her online. Loving our local neighbors does not require such extreme Luddite discipline. I hear you, and, on a good day, I even agree with you. Modern technology is not unraveling our ability to love our neighbors, but it is changing the places that make it possible to even have such a thing as neighbors.

Heading to Ford Heights without a car, cell phone, or computer worried us. We were concerned that our newly wireless life would isolate us rather than unite us with our neighbors. We were already odd enough as privileged outsiders led by visions of community, reconciliation, and kinship. Why add more "weird" to the package?

Our fears were quickly allayed. Neighbors questioned our lack of a television, but our other great technological sacrifices went unnoticed. We do not stand out. In Ford

Chico Fajardo-Heflin is an artist, dishwasher, and storyteller. He and his wife, Tatiana, currently share their home with two neighborhood teenagers. You cannot follow Chico on Twitter, but you can follow Jesus over to your next-door neighbor's house.

Heights, cars, tablet computers, and internet access are still luxuries. About a third of the people in our town don't own a car, and those who do must often share it with households of, say, seven. Computers can be spotted in less than half of our neighbors' homes, and internet access isn't a given. Smartphones are growing more common but are not pillars of daily life. I have yet to see an Apple Watch. The results of choices that made us seem radical to those outside Ford Heights are simply part of ordinary life for those in the neighborhood.

We are one lively, semidysfunctional family . . . and I love it.

What stands out to us about Ford Heights, however, is how well everyone knows one another. In the neighborhood, there is no such thing as a stranger. You are family, friend, or enemy – but never unknown. Walk down any street in the summer, and you're likely to find young mothers gossiping on front stoops, image-conscious teens flaunting their new shoes, and hordes of kids romping around. This sort of intimacy has its downsides ("Everybody be up in each other's business," as locals say), but mostly it is a gift.

Those who live in communities like Ford Heights know what I am talking about. Neighbors watch each other's kids. Lawnmowers are shared. Cousins and second cousins live across the street from each other. We are one lively, semidysfunctional family . . . and I love it.

This sort of close-knit village life was new for me. Prior to moving to Ford Heights, all my attempts at following the commandment to "love your neighbor as yourself" were in the context of sprawling suburbs or trendy urban neighborhoods. I marched in antiwar demonstrations, purchased fair-trade goods, and helped throw potlucks for homeless folks downtown. But any engagement with my actual next-door neighbors was conspicuously absent. How was I supposed to love my neighbors as myself when I hardly saw them? It doesn't seem possible in the transient, anonymous life found in most suburbs and cities.

Things are different in Ford Heights. With rowdy basketball games clogging the roads and kids always knocking on the door, loving one's neighbor becomes as simple and natural as attending a birthday party down the street.

Why is it that most suburbs and cities are random collections of strangers while places like Ford Heights are intimate communities? It occurs to me that the "localizing effect" Tatiana and I experienced as a result of our disconnection from modern technology has been at work in Ford Heights for years.

Our town's relative lack of access to modern technology has shielded it from what has turned much of North America into an anonymous society. In places like Ford Heights, the high cost of air travel has kept people from spreading out, allowing vast family trees to take root and inhabit a single place. Limited access to cars means options for shopping are restricted to what's in walking distance (the corner store) and not how far one can drive (the mall). And the fact that not everyone owns internet-connected devices translates into neighbors spending more time with friends in town than on Facebook.

I do not mean to romanticize my town's poverty. Rather, there seems to be a direct connection between the amount of technology a community adopts and its ability to maintain a close-knit social fabric. Because its residents are unable to afford the new American dream, Ford Heights has (mostly) bypassed the technological nightmare that comes with it.

The preservation of neighborhood life was not the reason Tatiana and I began to move away from modern technology, but it is surely one of the primary reasons we continue to do so. Neglected ghettos and dying rural towns are some of the last places left in North America where the greatest commandment can still be practiced with one's actual neighbors. But as corporations find ways to make their latest gadgets more affordable and advertisers continue to seduce young imaginations, the gift of a local life that so many of us here cherish hangs in the balance. The loneliness and anonymity that has struck so many cities and suburbs has begun to creep into Ford Heights. Television already keeps far too many residents inside, and too often neighbors choose YouTube over pickup basketball games.

We're not naïve enough to think our household's decision to stay offline and on the ground will do much to stop the technological invasion that is bound to come, but we love Ford Heights' block parties too much to be willing to give up the fight just yet. ➤

Why I Am Not Going to Buy a Computer

• • • • • • • • • • • • • WENDELL BERRY • • • • • • • • • • • •

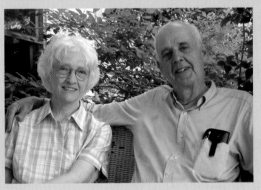

Like almost everybody else, I am hooked to the energy corporations, which I do not admire. I hope to become less hooked to them. In my work, I try to be as little hooked to them as possible. As a farmer, I do almost all of my work with horses. As a writer, I work with a pencil or a pen and a piece of paper.

My wife types my work on a Royal standard typewriter bought new in 1956 and as good now as it was then. As she types, she sees things that are wrong and marks them with small checks in the margins. She is my best critic because she is the one most familiar with my habitual errors and weaknesses. She also understands, sometimes better than I do, what ought to be said. We have, I think, a literary cottage industry that works well and pleasantly. I do not see anything wrong with it.

What would a computer cost me? More money, for one thing, than I can afford, and more than I wish to pay to people whom I do not admire. But the cost would not be just monetary. It is well understood that technological innovation always requires the discarding of the "old model" – the "old model" in this case being not just our old Royal standard, but my wife, my critic, my closest reader, my fellow worker. Thus (and I think this is typical of present-day technological innovation), what would be superseded would be not only something, but somebody. In order to be technologically up-to-date as a writer, I would have to sacrifice an association that I am dependent upon and that I treasure. ➤

Wendell and Tania Berry, 2010

Source: *What Are People For?: Essays* (Berkeley: Counterpoint, 1990), 170–171. Copyright © 1990, 2010 by Wendell Berry. Reprinted by permission of Counterpoint Press.

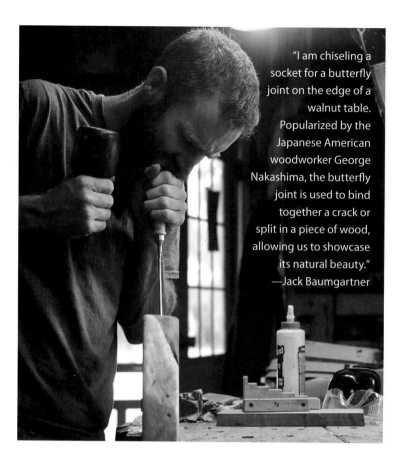

"I am chiseling a socket for a butterfly joint on the edge of a walnut table. Popularized by the Japanese American woodworker George Nakashima, the butterfly joint is used to bind together a crack or split in a piece of wood, allowing us to showcase its natural beauty."
—Jack Baumgartner

The Perfect Tool

On a Kansas farm, Jack and Amy Baumgartner are crafting a family.

SUSANNAH BLACK

Jack Baumgartner starts his day at 4:30. His wife and four children are still asleep, and early on a November morning, outside his tin-roofed house on the plains near Wichita, Kansas, it's still dark. But there's a lot to do. "Downstairs," he says, "I start the hot water for coffee. I stir the coals in the wood stove we heat our home with, remove some ashes, and place two mulberry logs on the embers to ignite. This is priestly work and an art near to my heart,

maintaining a fire for my family. It is a part of my worship."

Baumgartner, age forty-two, is a farmer. He's also a woodworker, painter, musician, and puppeteer. "I have invested a lot in each area over time," he told the writer Elizabeth Duffy in a 2014 interview, "so I feel comfortable in each realm." This November morning, he brings his coffee and homemade bagel – his wife makes them – into the insulated garage

Photography courtesy of Jack Baumgartner

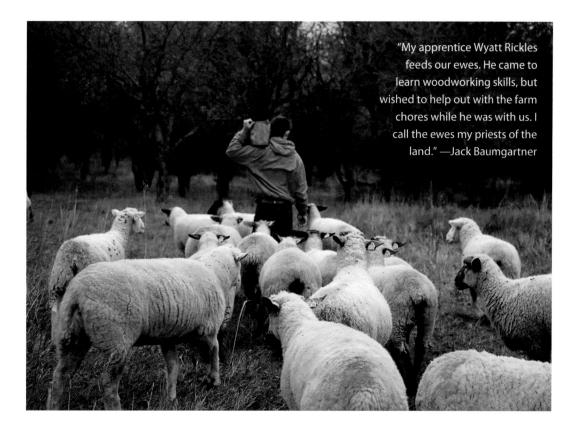

"My apprentice Wyatt Rickles feeds our ewes. He came to learn woodworking skills, but wished to help out with the farm chores while he was with us. I call the ewes my priests of the land." —Jack Baumgartner

next to the house that he uses as a studio. He's working on a block of linoleum, carving an image: he's a printmaker as well. Some of these he sells from the Etsy shop that he and his wife use to market their goods: his prints and turned wooden bowls, her goat's-milk soap.

Until a couple of years ago, just before their fourth child was born, Amy, Jack's wife, was working as a Presbyterian minister in Wichita. Jack was running the farm and his growing woodworking business and homeschooling the kids (the oldest is ten). But she left her job so that, as he describes it, "she could be a mom, finally." It wasn't easy. "As we were making the transition to losing the bulk of our financial security," he says, "there was a lot of questioning from family and acquaintances. 'How are you guys going to survive?'"

The answer to that question is the story of their days: they're living on a patchworked domestic economy that takes a great deal of human energy, a great deal of commitment, and a great deal of creativity. The woodworking brings in the most money – later on that day, he'll finish a custom poker table he's making for a lodge in Montana – but the farming supplies much of the food. Before he can get to work on the poker table, his chores include checking the health of an ailing ewe-lamb; Amy milks the goats; the children collect eggs.

He feeds the pigs, stepping carefully over the electric fence, racing to reach the feeding pans before the pigs reach him. "I have to win," he says, "or I can't get the food past their greedy heads and bodies smashing into my legs and crowded around the plastic tubs. The kids

Susannah Black is a contributing editor to Plough *and has written for publications including* First Things, Front Porch Republic, Mere Orthodoxy, *and* The American Conservative. *She lives in New York City.*

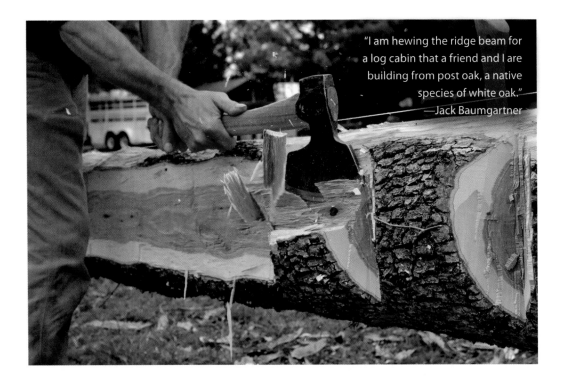

"I am hewing the ridge beam for a log cabin that a friend and I are building from post oak, a native species of white oak."
—Jack Baumgartner

don't get to feed the pigs unless we have spoiled vegetables from my friend's farm down the road. Then they hurl them over the fence at the pigs, laughing."

It's a way of life that integrates work and family. "I once read about the effects of the industrial revolution on families," says Baumgartner, "about how homes were once the primary place of industry; maybe a shop on the ground floor and living quarters above. This was the playing field where life happened. Home was a perpetual bustle of life and community. I work long hours, but I am home and my children and my wife have access to me and I to them. We live together, not apart."

A key aspect of that living-together has to do with choosing what technology to use in their household. To characterize Baumgartner and his wife as anti-technology is to miss the point entirely: technology – tools and their right use – is something that Baumgartner regards as a great good. This good is a theme to which he returns again and again. He refers to his tools as "the technology of my worship.

The axe is the perfect tool, as a woodworker. It is *the* tool. It is tool. Every woodworking tool is resting there in the axe waiting to be born." He hopes, he says, to be a craftsman in the line of Bezalel, the Old Testament character, who "fashioned so much for the tabernacle, making the sacred things that were part of the 'technology' of worship of his God for his community. Bezalel is a paradigm of an artisan of broad experience – he could work in many trades and arts with skill worthy of God's tabernacle."

Working with tools is the crucial way that he feeds his "hunger to see and participate with more of God in every particle of everything." The technology he prefers does not insulate him from the concrete world but embeds him in it. He's drawn to "thinking about and using 'old' technology," he says on his website, "where I can really see and feel the principles at work. Where I can experience the relationship of design and purpose in my hands. The partnership of a wedge and lever in a well-made axe is filled with grace and wonder. So it goes with

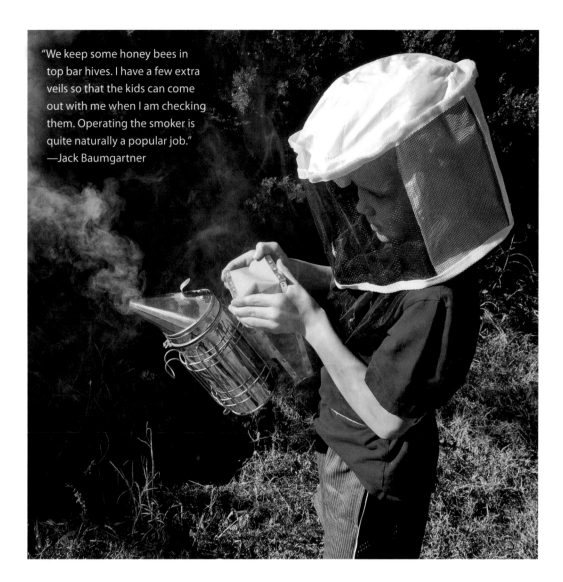

"We keep some honey bees in top bar hives. I have a few extra veils so that the kids can come out with me when I am checking them. Operating the smoker is quite naturally a popular job."
—Jack Baumgartner

many tools: a moldboard plow, a scythe, or a block and tackle."

Baumgartner rejects the separation between the theoretical and practical, between knowledge and know-how. "I can't stand education I can't do something with," he says. "I can only study so much before I am outside working again, putting things into application. I am glad I am seeing those traits in my children. You read about something, then you try to build it yourself, or make it happen. We can do darn near anything around here with tools and knowledge. Everyone who comes to our farm knows that we love tools, and knows that my kids learn to use them as soon as they are able."

The skills that he's passing down to his children are not separable from the faith that he is likewise passing down. Raised Presbyterian, he says that his father's and grandfathers' presence in his life led him to have a strong sense of God as a present father. "My granddad was a gifted woodcarver," he explains, "and I spent a lot of time with him in his workshop. My dad, too, is a builder and carver, so the weekends and summers were often spent making things."

Having received skills and faith from others, Baumgartner feels accountable to pass them on. On one November evening, he told

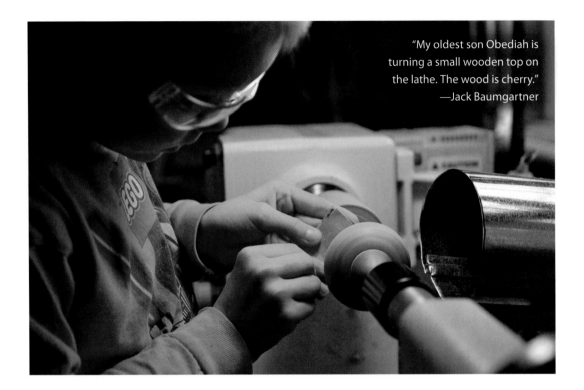

"My oldest son Obediah is turning a small wooden top on the lathe. The wood is cherry."
—Jack Baumgartner

me, his ten-year-old son "turned a carving mallet out of Osage orange on the lathe. He was constantly calling me over to talk about all of the details he was noticing in the wood, all the nuances of its beauty. He finished the piece with excellence, leaving no rough spots, no tool marks, and no scratches from the heavier grits of sandpaper. He is no master yet, far from it, but he is on the path that will take him there if he wants to go."

Baumgartner is also passing these skills on to those beyond his family. Recently, a young man contacted him, an aspiring woodworker looking for mentoring. He's moved into their household for the duration of his informal apprenticeship. "I am passing on to one who is hungry for them lessons I learned from my dad and granddad, and my own lessons as well. I am teaching him how to hold his body when he saws, how to be conscious of his grip when he concentrates. How to intuitively feel when a tool is square as it meets the wood."

Despite his commitment to traditional tools, Baumgartner is no Luddite. When his youngest son was twenty-one days old, he began to show symptoms of a lymphatic disorder. Modern medicine saved the baby's life. Meanwhile, Baumgartner's father is on the list for an organ transplant. "I watched modern medicine save the two living bookends of my family," he says. "And I was confident that I was watching God display his goodness, and I was confident that I was missing a lot of the picture. But the line of stewardship, I could see."

This line of stewardship is the mandate that we have to work in the material world. God can perform healing miracles, as he can perform miracles of the multiplication of bread, of fish, of wine. But he doesn't always do so. Baumgartner believes that "God invited us to be a part of the world He created and [in which he] hid away countless treasures for us to unlock and grow."

He and his wife have not made a single,

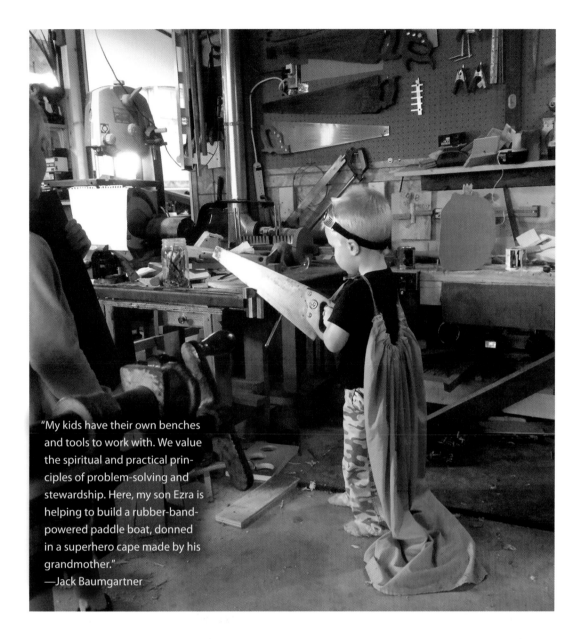

"My kids have their own benches and tools to work with. We value the spiritual and practical principles of problem-solving and stewardship. Here, my son Ezra is helping to build a rubber-band-powered paddle boat, donned in a superhero cape made by his grandmother."
—Jack Baumgartner

ideologically driven choice to reject something called "modern technology." Instead, they've made a series of choices to do and make and play and work together. "We cure our own hams and bacon. We don't take vacations. We go into debt to buy a farm. We let our children work with knives. We get shit on our hands and feet and track it in the house. We grow wheat and harvest it with sickles and scythes, thresh it and winnow it by hand, grind it by hand. We break lots of things. We fix lots of things, but not as many as we break. We sing, we dance, we fight. We are like the rest of the whole world. We grow our own food and we like Skittles."

They are crafting their family, their days, to make something of lasting value. And they're attempting to choose, in each case, the right tool for the job. ⤳

Read the full interview with Jack Baumgartner at plough.com/baumgartner.

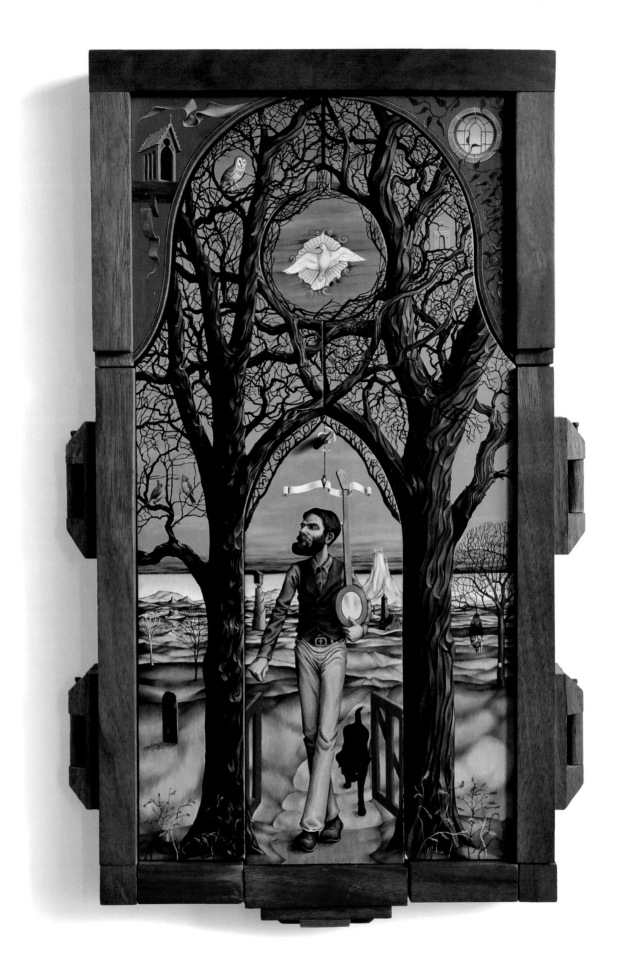

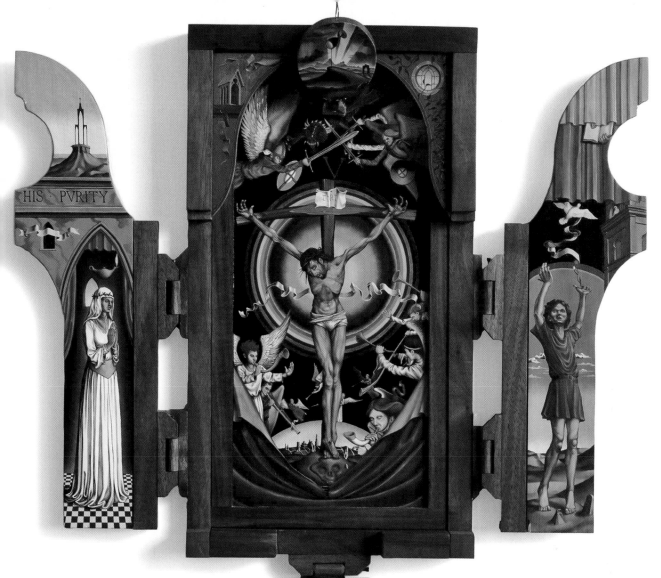

Jack Baumgartner,
Go On, Inner Man, triptych

"I began this painting while living as a hermit in Kansas. By the time it was finished it had grown into a wedding gift to my wife. The original premise was the contrast between the outer man in the physical world and the inner man in the spiritual world – and the reconciliation between the two through Christ's sacrifice. It also embodies my own journey from hermit-hood and isolation to marriage and community.

"The front panel *(left)* is a self portrait of me and my dog, Doc, walking through 'The Gate of Hearing and Walking.' (The branches over the gate spell that title out.) While I lived in the dormant landscape behind me, my daily walks were my prayers to God.

"The inside panel shows the crucifixion, with the cup of Christ's blood being poured over the earth. That is me worshiping at the foot of the cross, the Bride of Christ praying on the left, and a young King David dancing on the right.

"I have always been deeply influenced by Northern European Renaissance art and the spiritual visions of those painters. You can see the influences of Bruegel, Grünewald, and a little Bosch in this altarpiece."

—Jack Baumgartner

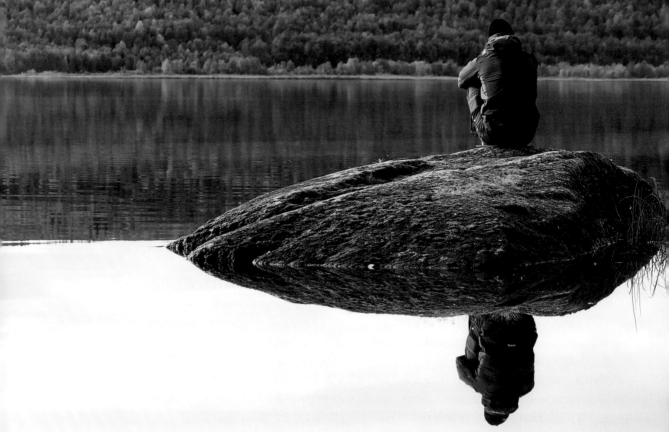

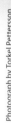

Endangered Habitat

Why the soul needs silence

STEPHANIE BENNETT

*Just as we protect endangered natural habitats, so we must preserve
the space that allows both speech and the soul to flourish.*

Silence is disappearing. It's disappearing
because we're being trained to hate it.

Accustomed as most of us are to
constant motion and busyness, many of
us structure our days to avoid silence at all
costs. For one, it's awkward. When the door
of an elevator shuts on a group of strangers,
the compulsion to fill the space with sound
is nearly palpable. Silence is "dead air," to
borrow a term from the radio business for any
gap in sound lasting longer than a second.

Only today, it's not just audible noises – the
beeps and vibrations of our various personal
devices – that break silence. Far more conse-
quential is the onslaught of images and words
with which they daily violate the interior
silence of our souls.

This rarely bothers most people, since
silence, as well as being uncomfortable, can be
fearsome. Leaving us alone with our thoughts,
it forces us to address matters we often sidestep
in our active outer lives. "Frightening," "lonely,"

"depressing" – these are just a few of the descriptors I come across when grading the essays of my students after asking them to fast from electronic media for twenty-four hours. The titles of their essays are telling: "My Day from Hell," or "Death – take me now!"

Over twelve years of assigning this exercise, I've noticed students have found it increasingly difficult to successfully stick out the digital fast. For many, severing the link to their main conduit of information causes something near emotional pain. Yet those who persevere through the initial feelings of loss often report an unexpected breakthrough. Some say they attain moments of great clarity and awareness; others find themselves gaining an almost ecstatic creativity. It's not uncommon for students to feel the urge to pray.

All the same, few if any of my students feel urged to make digital fasting a regular part of life. I suspect this has to do with the third and most powerful reason we avoid silence: it presents us with the stark realization of our own frailty, failure, and eventual death. Loosed from the concerns of the workaday world, we can feel purposeless and adrift, aware of the short span of human consciousness we call life. For those who are older, silence may push the lost dreams of youth to the forefront of the imagination. We live, we die; the cycle continues. Who wants to be confronted with the harshness of that reality?

Yet this is a medicine we need. Silence does the deep work that speech cannot accomplish. Through its discipline, we come to better understand our own thoughts and motivations. We find ourselves relating more cohesively to our world and to others. We can gain a stronger grasp of what it means to be human.

That's why it matters that silence is endangered. This state of affairs hasn't come upon us all at once – even before the Industrial Revolution, technologies such as print were transforming and increasing the flow of information, with profound effects on the interior lives of human beings. Yet the revolution in digital media has made the loss of silence not just one reason for concern among many, but an acute threat – and indeed, an accomplished fact for most humans alive today.

The huge increase in information flooding our brains makes dramatic new demands on their capacity for mental processing, which in turn may help explain why stress and related anxiety disorders are on the rise.[1] "Information/action imbalance" is what the educator Neil Postman called this growing phenomenon in a book written in 1985, years before the internet was widely available.[2] Postman hypothesized that the ratio between information received and a person's ability to act on that information creates psychological stress.

Postman, in turn, built on the work of Jacques Ellul, a French philosopher and historian writing two decades earlier. Already then, Ellul foresaw the implications of big data for the interior life: "Like a fish's perfect adaptation to its water environment, we are enveloped in data, absorbed into a mono-dimensional world of stereotypes and slogans, and integrated into a homogenous whole by the machinery of conformity."

Today this "machinery of conformity" permeates every niche of our culture. Nearly five billion people use mobile phones,[3] and

> Silence does the deep work that speech cannot accomplish.

Stephanie Bennett, PhD, is fellow for student engagement and professor of communication and media ecology at Palm Beach Atlantic University. She is author of several books, including The Poet's Treasure *(Wild Flower Press, 2016), a work of fiction about the future of community.*

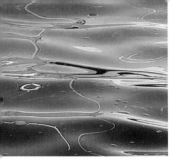

Digital devices corrode the ability to communicate face to face.

computerization affects virtually all areas of human life, from media and medicine to retail and relationships. From an economic point of view, of course, the deluge of largely unnecessary information is a boon; entire new industries have sprung up to capture, save, mine, and sell data on the information we consume. Yet, especially since the widespread adoption of social media, the human brain's remarkable filtering ability is showing signs of being overtaxed.

Simply put, the problem is internal noise. Noise is as different from speech as weeds are from flowers; if not brought under control, it can take over a whole landscape. Unceasing internal noise replaces the reflective space one needs to think, ponder, wonder, and pray. In his 2014 book *The End of Absence,* journalist Michael Harris chronicles what he terms "the end of empty space." He addresses the growing absence of silence and wonders if the next generation will find it more difficult to access solitude. "Will 'deep' conversation and solitary walks be replaced by an impoverished experience of text clouds?" he asks. "Will the soft certainty of earlier childhood be replaced by the restless idleness that now encroaches?" [4]

These are urgent questions if we're serious about preserving those elements of our humanness that make us distinct from machines. A regular measure of silence gives us a refreshed inner terrain. It affords us the opportunity to focus, not on our internal distractions, but on other people with whom we are in relationship. It helps us better use words and actions to communicate meaning. It allows intimacy.

Sherry Turkle, an MIT professor researching in the field of technology and social science, argues that digital devices, far from connecting us with others, actually corrode the ability to communicate face to face. Turkle's 2015 book, *Reclaiming Conversation,* points to a decreasing ability to carry on complex conversations. In her view, the first step toward reclaiming the art of conversation is to regain the solitude that we have let ebb away from daily life: "Without solitude we can't construct a stable sense of self. Yet children who grow up digital have always had something external to respond to. When they go online, their minds are not wandering, but rather are captured and divided." [5]

Essential to both conversation and to intimacy is the sound of the human voice. After all, a human being is not a brain in a vat; we are people with a mind and soul in a body, and that body speaks – uniquely, audibly, and replete with meaning. The presence of the word has a significance that goes beyond the mere functional need to convey a message, as the linguist Walter J. Ong recognized:

> The word itself is both interior and exterior: it is, as we have seen, a partial exteriorization of an interior seeking another interior. The primary physical medium of the word – sound – is itself an exteriorization of a physical interior, setting up reverberations in other physical interiors. [6]

Thus, when two people sit down to speak with each other, they naturally tend to enter into relationship with one another. When we cease to use our gift of speech as our primary way of knowing – deferring to more remote systems of mediating reality such as writing, texting, or seeing – we place another layer between our external and internal knowing.

Superficial relationships are those that stay on the periphery of each individual; the intimate ones are born from a desire to mine the riches of another's soul. Our ability to know

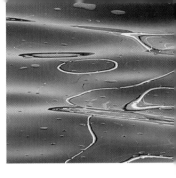

another person is directly related to our ability to be with that person – within earshot – communicating via the spoken word rather than through the mere exchange of text on a page or a screen. The reality of this interiority comes sharply into view when we experience loneliness. Loneliness is born out of emotional distance from others and is one of the leading complaints from those struggling with depression.[7] The erosion of intimacy and emotional distance are often cited as key contributors in divorce court.

"It is one's voice that bespeaks presence."[8] Though the voice can admittedly also be heard through the telephone or a call app, these mediating devices drape a cloak of unknowing over conversation. The word spoken in the physical presence of another creates an opportunity to go beyond the substance of a message and enter the realm of mystery. Ellul explains:

> We are in the presence of an infinitely and unexpectedly rich tool, so that the tiniest phrase unleashes an entire polyphonic gamut of meaning. The ambiguity of language, even its ambivalence and its contradiction, between the moment it is spoken and the moment it is received, produces extremely intense activities. Without such activities, we would be ants or bees, and our drama and tragedy would quickly be dried up and empty. Between the moment of speech and the moment of reception are born symbol, metaphor, and analogy.[9]

Before electronic media, print, or writing, there was speech. From the cry of a newborn to the last words of one dying, there exists a link between being and speaking. Speech is the initial and primary means by which our thoughts and perceptions are mediated; the vocal mechanism creates an echo of the self reaching out to another person. This reverberating effect is what makes rich relationships possible.

The discipline of the well-spoken word depends, in turn, on silence. When it is absent from our daily lives, the power of our words is reduced and we are left with the scraps of language – acronyms, emojis, and downsized meaning. It's unsurprising, then, that the information age has renewed interest in the art of mindfulness. Scores of recent articles, for example, discuss the scientific rationale for meditation. The practice of silence for spiritual strength and mental clarity is of course hardly a novel discovery, but anchored in thousands of years of history.

Silence is a necessary counter to the relentless preoccupation of our multitasking minds – something that should provide a contrapuntal rhythm to the steady beat of our busy human brains. Just as we are wise to protect the earth's vulnerable woodlands from overdevelopment, so we must protect the sanctuary of our interior lives. Speech, relationships, the soul: they begin with, and are sustained by, silence. ⤳

We are in the presence of an infinitely and unexpectedly rich tool.

1. Neil Postman, *Amusing Ourselves to Death: Public Discourse in the Age of Show Business* (Viking Penguin, 1985).

2. Ibid.

3. Simon Kemp, "We are Social," *Global Overview, Special Reports*, January 24, 2017. *wearesocial.com*

4. Michael Harris, *The End of Absence* (Penguin, 2015), 39.

5. Sherry Turkle, *Reclaiming Conversation* (Penguin, 2015), 61.

6. Walter J. Ong, *The Presence of the Word* (University of Minnesota Press, 1967).

7. Steve Horsmon, "A Research-Based Approach to Strengthening Relationships," March 6, 2017, The Gottman Institute. *gottman.com*

8. Frank E. X. Dance, "Digitality's Debt to Speech," in *Explorations in Media Ecology*, vol. 7, no. 1, ed. Corey Anton (2002), 38.

9. Jacques Ellul, *The Humiliation of the Word*, trans. J. M. Hanks (Eerdmans, 1985), 19.

The Pen & the Keyboard

MARK BAUERLEIN

If you go online and type into the search box "Pelikan fountain pen 1950s," dozens of images pop up displaying vintage items for sale. They range in value, some as low as fifty dollars, gold nib and all. "Go out and buy one," I encourage the students in my classes and the teens and twenty-somethings in the audience when I give a lecture. "Tell your parents that you want an old fountain pen for Christmas or graduation."

I hold up a pen of my own and they gaze at it with some curiosity and amusement. When I exhort them to get one for themselves, they look quizzical at first, and then interested. Nobody had ever suggested this to them before, and it makes them reflect. It's as if a new character trait springs upon them and makes them ponder themselves in a new, more expansive way. A fancy pen of my own . . .

> The strangeness of handwriting is part of its advantage.

American youths are so enveloped in digital novelties that an old-fashioned implement wholly foreign to peer pressure and youth culture strikes them as a puzzle – but a compelling one. They do like the idea of a personal writing tool, though it never occurred to them before. A vintage pen signifies much more than just another tool, even to the tuned-in and logged-on Millennial.

The reason is simple. Consider one of the things you do with that pen: sign your name. A signature is a special action. It identifies a human being; more than that, it uniquely stands for him. It is individual. When you sign your name, you inscribe yourself. Nobody else can do it – only you. In fact, your signature has legal and binding status.

There we have the great distinction between the pen and the keyboard. When ten people type a sentence onto the screen, they all create the exact same thing. When they write identical words by hand, the material product varies with every writer. Every hand is singular, and so is each person's handwriting. When a twenty-year-old drops the keyboard and takes up the fountain pen, a wondrous individualization transpires. The keyboard "technologizes" them into users. There, they produce the same fonts. The pen characterizes them as distinct. They produce unique scripts.

And let's not reduce the value of handwriting to a decorative feature. Close the laptop and hand a Millennial a Mont Blanc or Parker or Visconti, and he will value more highly the art of writing. He will take his words more seriously. They will appear as his creation. He made those words, not

Mark Bauerlein is senior editor at First Things *and professor of English at Emory University, and has also served at the National Endowment for the Arts. His books include* The Pragmatic Mind: Explorations in the Psychology of Belief *(1997) and* The Dumbest Generation: How the Digital Age Stupefies Young Americans and Jeopardizes Our Future *(2008).*

a computer. The pen, thereby, becomes an extension of his sensibility. When he has a pen in his hand – especially a pen that was not mass-produced – he feels a heavier burden of self-expression. The individuality of his handwriting promotes the individuality of his writing. To compose a cliché with a Pelikan in hand is harder than to compose one on a Mac.

Of course, 21st-century youths look at handwriting as a clunky process, and the schools support them. Instruction in cursive writing has steadily disappeared from the elementary school curriculum. Now, when college students hand in their tests, teachers struggle to decipher the scratchings they submit.

But the strangeness of handwriting is part of its advantage. Its inefficiency affects students in just the way English teachers want. Young people do everything else with the keyboard, and when they write a paper on it the act blends with all the other messages they send in the day's communications. Writing by hand forces them into a plodding endeavor that won't yield to interruptions or accustomed habits of expression. When they compose on a computer, students are constantly deflected by emails or the ding of new text messages, and these diversions break the verbal flow. Nothing like that can happen with only a page in front of them. What the students take as an impoverishment is, in fact, an improvement.

And so I press them to acquire a pen, an old one that isn't like anybody else's. Most students come to college with little confidence in their writing abilities,[1] and freshman composition may be the most dreaded and disliked course in college. Students want to move on to business and pre-med and psychology, not prolong the drudgery of exposition. They know they aren't good at it, too (only 61 percent of entering students are even "college ready" for freshman English, according to ACT).[2] Every paper assignment makes them anxious, and they employ the customary tactics of coping. They consult websites for ideas, for instance, a web page that hands them an interpretation of an Emily Dickinson poem, and delay the work until the night before the paper is due. Then they open the laptop and pound out the sentences as fast as they can. Anything to avoid making the writing process a careful, deliberate, and expressive activity. It's too unpleasant.

But handwriting nudges them in another direction. It asks students to approach their writing not so much as a mechanical procedure but as a creative one, or at least an individual one. They will work harder to make their prose live up to the pen in their hand. All of them want the latest iPhone. The colleges they attend boast of cutting-edge technology. But all those tools are mass-produced. Kids who get an iPhone or tablet immediately set about customizing them. At the mall they browse the kiosks that display rows of cell phone cases in wild colors. They want to tailor their gear to their personality. The Digital Age promises to amplify their being – YouTube's original motto was "Broadcast Yourself" – but, in truth, it only delivers a horde of users with identical devices echoing one another in cyberspace.

Instead of joining the digital race, a youth with a sixty-year-old Parker Duofold simply draws it out of his pocket, unscrews the cap, opens the notebook, and begins scribbling. It's distinguished and it's fun. Most of all, for those of us who teach writing, not to mention the employers who complain about bad prose in the workplace, it leads the youths we want to improve to do just that, to write better sentences and paragraphs. ⇒

1. Kevin Eagan et al., "The American Freshman: National Norms Fall 2015" Higher Education Research Institute, UCLA, 2015. *heri.ucla.edu*

2. ACT, "The Condition of College and Career Readiness 2017," September 7, 2017. *act.org*

Meet a True Story

MICHAEL T. McRAY

Technology feeds our insatiable hunger for stories, but fails to satisfy our need for human connection. A boom in live storytelling could be changing that.

When I moved to Ireland for graduate school in 2012, Pádraig Ó Tuama, a leader of the Corrymeela Community, was the first person I met. As he drove me into the city from the airport, he invited me to the monthly storytelling event he and Paul Doran ran known as Tenx9 (pronounced "ten by nine"), where nine people had ten minutes each to tell a real story from their lives, based on a theme.

In the months I lived in Belfast, I attended every Tenx9, and when I returned to Nashville, I asked Pádraig and Paul if I could start a chapter back home. They agreed, and I ran the first event in September 2013, with another following every month since.

It didn't take long before people began noticing how popular live storytelling events

were becoming. Events like Tenx9 have popped up around town and around the country. People want storytelling, in part because of a longing for human connection. In this technological age, we've become increasingly digitally connected and simultaneously locally estranged. We're losing much of the intimacy of intentional human connection, trading it for constant connectivity, availability, and impersonal comments sent to "someone" "somewhere else."

At Tenx9, we try to cultivate human connection by being a place where ordinary people tell ordinary stories. Alongside silly and delightful stories, you can hear stories of pain and struggle. At the first Nashville event, the theme was "Journey," and a friend of mine shared a story about an incredible biking adventure he took with his dad. The audience

---

Michael T. McRay is the founder and curator of Tenx9 Nashville Storytelling. He lectures at Lipscomb University and is the author of Letters from "Apartheid Street" *and* Where the River Bends. *michaelmcray.com*

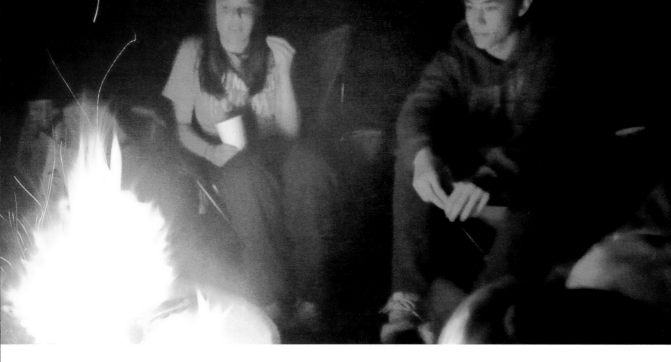

Photographs by Jason Bennett

smiled and laughed and relaxed. The very next story was also about a father, but one quite different. The storyteller told of her turbulent relationship with her dad, of always wanting to feel loved by him. She told how that longing began to mask itself with anger. And then she shared about the day she got a call that her father had been found dead in his garage, car exhaust filling his vehicle, and a goodbye note left behind – for her.

An Irish proverb says, "It is in the shelter of each other that the people live." We can give shelter to each other by telling stories of what it means to be human, and by listening generously. I've worked in prisons, in education, and in healthcare advocacy. In all these contexts, one of the clearest dilemmas facing people is the inability to listen to and empathize with others who see the world differently. We are quick to unfriend, unfollow, and police anyone who creates dissonance in our echo chambers; we're like hawks, soaring over the landscape of social discourse to look for anything and anyone we need to swoop down and silence. We seem to be listening only for variations on anthems we already love or for the choruses of songs we hope to mute. Listening with

patience, listening for the sake of learning, is becoming a lost art.

Stories against Fear

A friend who's a neurobiologist once told me the brain automatically categorizes people into "similar and dissimilar." The "similar" ones we trust quickly, the "dissimilar" ones we don't. Our brains, for survival's sake, feed this persistent paranoia that unless we are the same, we are in danger. Storytelling is one way we escape this thinking.

> **Storytelling is one way we escape from us-versus-them thinking.**

In Northern Ireland, I met a remarkable English woman named Jo Berry. On October 12, 1984, Jo's world exploded when her father, a British MP, was killed by an IRA bomb at the Grand Hotel in Brighton, England. Two months later, she serendipitously shared a taxi with a man from Belfast whose brother had been in the IRA before being killed by a British soldier. "We should have been enemies," Jo told me, "but instead we spoke of a world where people didn't kill each other." She left knowing she needed to "bridge the divide . . . to try to understand those that killed" her father.

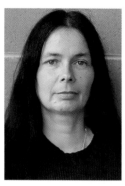

Jo Berry

Photograph from the Irish Times/PA

During the next fifteen years, Jo told her story at conferences on forgiveness. She says this helped her heal – and, in hearing the stories of others, she even began to understand why someone might join the IRA.

In 1999, her life changed again when Patrick Magee, the man responsible for her father's death, walked out of prison as part of the Good Friday Agreement. One year later, Jo's friend arranged a meeting. When Patrick walked through the door, Jo shook his hand and thanked him for coming. During the next three hours, they talked alone. "I didn't want to blame him," she said to me. "I wanted him to open up. I needed to hear his story." Initially, though, all she heard was "political justification." Uninterested in hearing Patrick justify her father's murder, she planned to end the meeting. But then Patrick said something different: "I don't know what to say anymore. I don't know who I am. Can I hear your rage? What can I do to help you?" The conversation had shifted, and Jo knew this wouldn't be their only meeting.

As they parted ways, Patrick apologized "with great feeling" for killing her father. Jo told me Patrick was "disarmed" by her empathy; it changed him. When Jo arrived home, she felt disoriented. "I've just met the enemy," she thought, "and I've seen his humanity." Now what?

To date, Patrick and Jo have spoken together over a hundred times, all over the world. He is no longer just the IRA bomber who killed her father; he is also the friend who teaches her how to solve cryptic crossword puzzles on planes.

Dismantling our enemies requires at least three steps: proximity, curiosity, and humility. We must be close enough to listen, curious enough to want to know more than we already do about the other's story, and humble enough to wonder if perhaps we've been wrong about the other all along. If we can, like Jo, get close enough to hear the story of our enemy, we may be able to subvert the narrative of fear that has controlled us for far too long.

Inhabit Another's Story

Recently, I've begun working with Narrative 4, a nonprofit that runs empathy-building programs all over the world. The core methodology is a story exchange, where paired participants tell their partner a true story from their life. Their partner listens deeply to the story. Then, when the participants regroup, each person tells their partner's story in *first-person pronouns,* as if that story happened to them. Former United Nations Secretary General Ban Ki-Moon said that the world is suffering from an "empathy gap." Narrative 4 is trying to address this gap.

In early September, I collaborated with a local nonprofit to bring together a group of twelve Christians, Muslims, and Jews to participate in such a story exchange. Gathering in the home of a Palestinian Christian, I watched a white Christian woman inhabit the story of a brown Muslim woman. I watched a Jewish man give his story to a Muslim man to tell. Afterward, each of the twelve expressed surprise at how they had learned to connect and empathize with each other. One woman said she felt freer, as well: hearing someone else tell her story lifted the burden of carrying it alone. At the end of our time together, another participant said, "This was possibly the closest experience of encountering the divine in the world that I've ever had."

These are gifts we can give each other when we listen well. When we soak ourselves in the story of another person enough to retell it, we begin to subvert the all-too-common pattern of listening to others only to craft our next retort. We start to see each other as humans rather than simply ideological positions to be out-argued.

Cracks of Hope

While practicing empathetic storytelling and listening can be difficult with a friend, doing so with your enemy is even harder. During recent storytelling projects in Israel, Palestine, Northern Ireland, and South Africa, I interviewed dozens of people who have done just that. One of the people I met was Bassam Aramin.

Bassam is a middle-aged Palestinian man who, at age seventeen, was sentenced to seven years in Israeli prison after a group of his friends threw grenades at Israeli soldiers. (No one was injured.) On October 1, 1987, around one hundred Israeli soldiers entered the youth wing of the prison as part of a military exercise. The 120 inmates were forced to strip, then beaten in a gauntlet formation. When they seized Bassam, he resisted and was taken into a side room for a more severe beating. As the soldiers struck him repeatedly, some were smiling. Yet at that moment, he remembered a film he had watched about the mass murder of Jews in the Nazi death camps. Strangely, at that moment he felt empathy for his enemies.

Afterward, while Bassam was still in prison, one of his Israeli jailers began conversations with him, challenging him on the story Bassam believed about his history, politics, and people. As the jailer and Bassam each told his understanding of the conflicted story of Israelis and Palestinians, Bassam hoped to convince the man to his way of thinking; I suspect the jailer hoped for the opposite. After a while, the jailer started bringing Bassam coffee – an attempt to provide some dignity and a sign of growing respect, or at least less disdain.

Some years later, after Bassam was free, he began meeting with former soldiers to exchange stories and hear different points of view, meetings that eventually led to the creation of Combatants for Peace. "I started to learn the other side," he told me. "Then I began to see the soldiers in the checkpoints not as targets. For the first time, I started to look at their faces. . . . The change starts in yourself. Rumi said, 'Yesterday I was clever, so I started to change the world. Today I am wise, so I start to change myself.'"

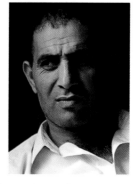

Bassam Aramin

In 2007, an Israeli soldier shot and killed Bassam's ten-year-old daughter, Abir, as she came home from school. Bassam's response to his daughter's killing was remarkable: he went to graduate school to study the Holocaust, hoping to better understand the history of his Jewish neighbors. Today Bassam is a spokesperson for Parents Circle–Families Forum, an organization of Israelis and Palestinians who have lost family members in the conflict.

> **If we can get close enough to hear the story of our enemy, we may be able to subvert the narrative of fear.**

These are the kinds of stories that can save us from succumbing to fear of the other. They subvert the narrative of the dangerous difference between "us" and "them." Rami Elhanan, the Israeli leader of the Parents Circle–Families Forum, whose fourteen-year-old daughter, Smadar, was killed by a Palestinian suicide bomber, once said to me, "We bang our heads against this very high wall of hatred and fear that divides these two nations. And we put cracks in it, cracks of hope." ➤

To learn more about Bassam Aramin's and Jo Berry's work, visit cfpeace.org *and* buildingbridgesforpeace.org.

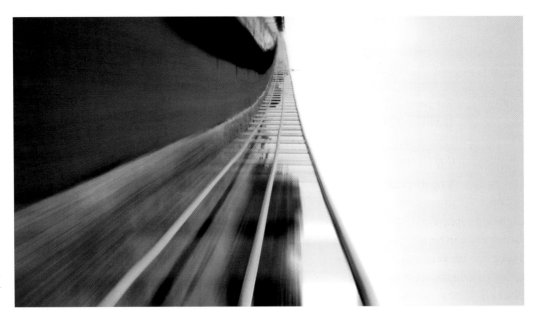

Photograph courtesy of turkletom

Tom Turkle,
Rollercoaster

A poem for my son about grace

"All of my heroes sit up straight." —*Gregory Alan Isakov*

My son slouches when he walks,
shoulders rounded, chin jutted
forward, his self moving slow
and savvy like Cecil the Turtle,
outwitting Bugs Bunny at every

turn. If the boy knew to say,
"Ain't I a stinka?" I bet he would.
In the church he sits, shoulder
blades pinned to the pew, enough
room between the seat and his lower

back to place a small child
or a couple of Eucharist plates.
At the altar of the rollercoaster,
the disembodied voice whispers,
"put your head back against the seat" –

the lap bar requiring our bodies
to obey 90 degrees before
we are launched 65 mph in fewer
than three seconds, and I grin,
my face flattening voluntarily

with glee as my son's back is straight
and his chin parallel with the earth
that is now hundreds of feet below
him, his eyes directed in front –
to seek the next turn or drop or twist

with hope with hope with faith with love,
I hope. He is forced into this position,
yes, I see that, and his shoulders
will curve again as the earth curves,
as the turtle's shell curves, keeping

him safe for now, but he did love
the ride, even when it broke
his wishes his routine his desires
and flattened him to its will.
Even then. Especially then.

JACOB STRATMAN

Editors' Picks

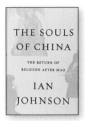

The Souls of China:
The Return of Religion After Mao
Ian Johnson
(Pantheon)

A century of suppression failed
to snuff out the faith of the
Chinese people. While relatively few profess
membership in an organized religion – an
unpopular Western concept for many
Chinese – religious belief and practice are alive
and well. Almost one third of Chinese are
religious, with roughly 200 million Buddhists
and Daoists, 60 million Protestants, 25 million
Muslims, and 10 million Catholics – with
another 175 million still following at least some
ancient Daoist or folk-religion practices.

Today, this book suggests, the number of
faithful is exploding as people look for meaning
and a moral compass. "A lot of us aren't poor
anymore, and yet we're still unhappy. We
realize there's something missing and that's a
spiritual life," one person tells the author.

Johnson, who has lived in China and
studied its religions since the early 1980s,
writes compellingly for one so knowledgeable.
The book is amazingly personal: it follows
families representing each faith through their
history and daily life to uncover deeply held
values and beliefs.

Mao Zedong's "Cultural Revolution"
crackdown on religion is well known, but the
destruction of temples and churches started
earlier, with the late emperors and the Nation-
alists also suppressing traditional Chinese
religion in hopes of moving their country
into the modern age. Mao sought to replace
religion with the cult of Mao. But, as Johnson
puts it succinctly, "there was one problem with
Mao as a living god: he died."

Persecution drove faith underground and
actually may have served to finally sever the
ancient link between state and religion. Now,
after three decades of relative openness, the
current government may try to rein in this
latest spiritual renewal or to coopt it for political purposes – but the tenacity of faith in China
over the last decades suggests that such efforts
are unlikely to succeed.

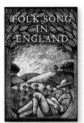

Folk Song in England
Steve Roud
(Faber & Faber)

It's easy to lament the
disappearance of old cultural
traditions, folk singing among
them. As we've turned away from the hearth of
communal music to our earbuds and personal
playlists, are we losing the variegated wealth of
folk song and music? In *Folk Song in England*,
Steve Roud asks a different question: Is there
even such a thing as a folk song? It's a question he takes over 700 pages to answer. Well
researched enough to satisfy the scholar but
lively enough to draw in the general reader, the
book traces the genealogy of folk music. When
arguing what makes a song a folk song, previous scholars typically focused on provenance.
Only songs with histories so long that they
disappeared into the mist of a legendary past
deserved to make the cut. Roud takes a different tack: What makes a folk song is, essentially,
where and how it was sung, and how it was
handed down.

Regarding folk song today, Roud allows
himself a little optimism. Thanks, in part,
to digitization, there is more folk material
readily available than ever before. "We may
even be approaching a golden age of folk song

research," Roud notes, "if only we have the people to embrace it." Might we say the same about folk singing? Few may have the time or passion to pick up folk song scholarship, but most of us can pick up a tune.

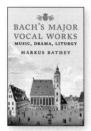

Bach's Major Vocal Works: Music, Drama, Liturgy
Markus Rathey
(Yale University Press)

An associate professor at Yale, Rathey has written an accessible guide to six of Bach's best-known choral works. The book is intended for "music lovers who want to read about a piece before going to a performance or before listening to a recording." If you haven't already, you would do well to make the *Christmas Oratorio* and *Saint Matthew's Passion* a regular part of your celebration of these church seasons.

Rathey focuses on a few recurring themes: the life of Jesus as celebrated in the liturgical calendar and, more surprisingly, Bach's clever use of love duets – a form popular in opera – to illustrate the relationship between Jesus and the believer. Rathey's insights into the love story between Christ and humanity, as described by early Lutheran theologians such as Johann Arndt, can open a new depth of understanding and appreciation for Bach's choral music. ⁓ *The Editors*

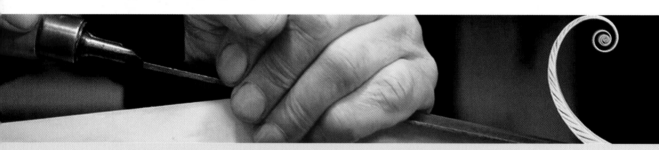

The Pencil Box

RICHARD LLEWELLYN

In Welsh author Richard Llewellyn's 1939 novel How Green Was My Valley, *the schoolboy Huw has just been given a finely crafted pencil box.*

There was no harm in that little box. A hundred years before, a craftsman in wood had put love into his job for all men to see in that little pattern of grained woods on the lid and round the sides. There was no need for him to spend those hours, for the box was made, but that pattern was his kiss of love, and I could see his hands passing over its smoothness, feeling its weight, having joy from the look and feel of it, and slow to let it pass into the hands of a buyer. . . .

Solomon never felt for his storehouse as I felt for that little box, and three men before me. To have pens, and pencils, and the tools of writing all your own, to see them and feel them in your fingers ready to do anything you tell them, to have them in a little house fit for them as good friends of yours, such is sweet pleasure, indeed, and never ending. For you open gently and take what you want, and careful in closing again, and you look at it before you start your work, and all the time a happy fullness inside you that sometimes will make you put out your hand to touch it as though to bless, so good you feel with it. God bless the craftsmen who give their fellow men such feelings even out of pieces of wood. ⁓

Source: *How Green Was My Valley* (Michael Joseph, 1939).

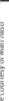

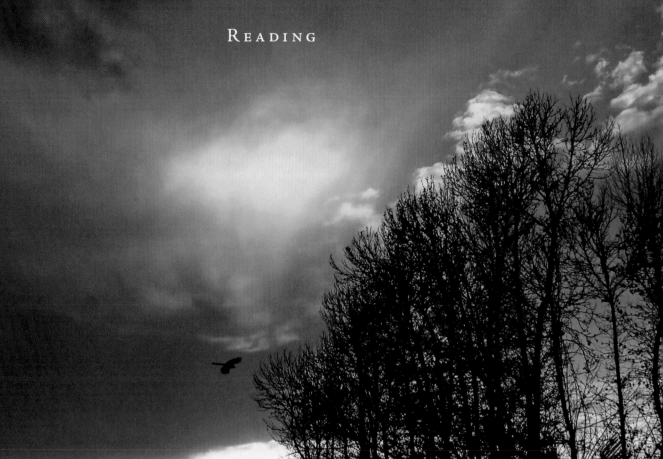

The Angels of Annunciation

ALFRED DELP

There always are angels of annunciation, speaking their message of good news into the midst of anguish, scattering their seed of blessing that will spring up one day in the midst of the night. They call us to hope. These are not yet the loud angels of rejoicing and fulfillment that come out into the open, like the angels of the first Christmas. Quiet, inconspicuous, they come into rooms and hearts as they did then. Quietly they bring God's questions and proclaim to us the wonders of God, for whom nothing is impossible.

From afar sound the first notes, not yet discernible as a song or melody. The new song of God's future is still far off and only just announced and foretold. But fulfillment is happening. It is occurring today. And tomorrow the angels will tell what has happened with loud, rejoicing voices, and we will know it and be glad. ➤

Alfred Delp (1907–1945) was a German Jesuit priest active in the resistance to Nazism who was executed in the aftermath of the failed 1944 July plot to overthrow Hitler.

Source: "The Shaking Reality of Advent," *Watch for the Light* (Plough, 2001).

Viktor Frankl

JASON LANDSEL

"Why do you not commit suicide?" With this question, psychiatrist Viktor Frankl offered his patients a key with which to unlock the chains of their afflictions. What, he was asking them, gave meaning to their lives? And his patients responded. Here was a doctor they could trust, whose theories were backed by personal experience.

Frankl was born March 26, 1905, in a Jewish section of Vienna, Austria. In 1921, at age sixteen, he gave his first lecture on "The Meaning of Life": he was already forming his philosophy of psychological healing through the discovery of meaning, an approach he would call Logotherapy.

Contrary to Sigmund Freud, Frankl affirmed that people are spiritual beings with free will, not just organisms responding reflexively to their environments. They are thus responsible for shaping their lives by choosing and working toward meaningful goals. The psychiatrist doesn't tell the patient what those goals should be, but helps the patient in a quest to discover them.

Frankl specialized in the treatment of depression and suicide at the University of Vienna, organizing a counseling program for students in 1930. He then began his own practice, but after the Nazi invasion of Austria in 1938 he was prohibited from treating non-Jewish patients. He became the director of a clinic for Jews where, at risk of his own life, he made false diagnoses to protect the mentally ill from euthanasia. It was under these conditions that he began writing his book *Ärztliche Seelsorge,* published in English as *The Doctor and the Soul.*

In 1939, Frankl could have immigrated to the United States, but chose to stay with his elderly parents. Three years later, he, his parents, and his wife, Tilly, were sent to the Theresienstadt concentration camp. Frankl and Tilly had married the previous year; the Nazis had forced her to abort their expected child.

Within half a year of arriving at the camp, Frankl's father died. Frankl, Tilly, and his mother were sent to Auschwitz in 1944. Frankl's mother was taken directly to the gas chamber. Tilly was moved to Bergen-Belsen, where she died in 1945; Frankl was sent to be a slave laborer in a sub-camp of Dachau.

At Dachau, Frankl started an underground psychiatric practice for suicidal prisoners: "We had to teach the despairing men that *it did not really matter what we expected from life, but rather what life expected from us,*" he explained later. The key to survival was to "listen to what your conscience commands you to do and to carry it out to the best of your knowledge." *

After the Allied forces liberated the camp, he made his way back to Vienna, where he learned of the death of his wife and his mother. For a year, he was close to despair. But in 1946 he returned to work. "Despair is suffering without meaning," he wrote. "If there is meaning in life at all, then there must be meaning in suffering."

That year, over the course of nine days, he dictated his best-known book, published in English as *Man's Search for Meaning.* At the heart of the meaning that we discover is love: "The salvation of man is through love and in love." ⤳

Jason Landsel is the artist for Plough's "Forerunners" *series, including the painting opposite.*

*Source: Viktor Frankl: Man's Search for Meaning (Beacon Press, 1959).